Hand Acupuncture Therapy

Written by Qiao Jinlin
Translated by Wang Tai

Foreign Languages Press   Beijing

First Edition   2002

Home Page:
http://www.flp.com.cn
E-mail Addresses:
info@flp.com.cn
sales@flp.com.cn

ISBN 7-119-03168-6
©Foreign Languages Press, Beijing, China, 2002

Published by Foreign Languages Press
24 Baiwanzhuang Road, Beijing 100037, China

Distributed by China International Book Trading Corporation
35 Chegongzhuang Xilu, Beijing 100044, China
P.O. Box 399, Beijing, China

Printed in the People's Republic of China

PREFACE

As a treasure of traditional Chinese medicine, hand acupuncture is a physiotherapy to prevent and treat diseases. The hand reveals — through changes of qi (vitality), color and outward appearance — physiological and pathological disturbances in the body. The same changes also reveal the cause and diagnosis of these diseases. Treatment for prevention or cure can then be applied by stimulating certain acupuncture points or areas of the hand through acupuncture, massage or other therapies.

Hand acupuncture therapy consists of two procedures: Diagnosis, through observing the hand; and treatment, through applying acupuncture and massage. The clinical practice of observing the hand can be traced to the Zhou Dynasty (c. 11th century-256 BC) where it was called palmistry or the holographic diagram of Jiu Gong (nine divisions) and Ba Gua (eight trigrams). Diagnosis through observing the hand developed further in the Qin and Han Dynasties (221 BC-AD 220). The publication of the ancient medical classics — such as *The Yellow Emperor's Canon of Medicine, Classic of Difficult Diseases* and so on — better defined and established the theories of Zangfu (internal organs) and Jingluo (meridians and collaterals). After that, observing the hand reached an even higher standard. Through this historical progression, hand acupuncture therapy developed into an important branch of traditional acupuncture.

Over the past 20 years — following the establishment and development of the biological holographic principle and holographic embryo theory — a diagnostic and therapeutic system developed for local acupuncture that combined the diagnostic diagram of the

i

hand's qi, color and appearance with the holographic embryo of the hand. Therefore, hand acupuncture therapy became increasingly scientific, systematic and objective. It acquired modern biological significance as it developed along a modern theoretical basis.

This book follows the history of hand acupuncture therapy as it developed to relate theories about the therapy; names, locations and identifying marks of acupuncture points and areas; and basic information on diagnosis. Further, the book discusses eight therapeutic methods and extensive clinical experiences involved in the treatment of over one hundred common diseases.

In writing the book, the author reviewed a vast amount of medical reference works, and received cordial encouragement from many specialists and scholars to whom he would like to express his heartfelt thanks. As for any errors that may appear — perhaps inevitably in a work of this scope — the author takes full responsibility and asks that diligent readers point them out so that they might be corrected in future editions.

Finally, the author hopes that this book will prove helpful to the many practitioners — both at home and abroad — of hand acupuncture therapy.

Qiao Jinlin
September 1998

CONTENTS

CHAPTER 1

INTRODUCTION

Section 1   Definition of Hand Acupuncture Therapy

What is hand acupuncture therapy? Before answering that question, let's first talk about something from common experience in daily life:

A toothache and its local swelling may have been caused by using the teeth to crack open too many melon seeds over a long period of time or it might have been induced by mental aggravation or anxiety. In any case, a common Chinese saying goes: "A toothache is not a serious illness, but the suffering it produces can drive a patient to death."

For those suffering a toothache, some concerned and knowledgeable people might recommend applying pressure to the Hukou point ("snuff-box," a depression between the first and second metacarpal bones of the palm) for two to three minutes to relieve the pain. Why? The explanation has a solid basis in medical theory. As mentioned in textbooks on Traditional Chinese Medicine, the Hegu (LI 4) point of the hand's Yangming large intestine meridian lies in the Hukou area. So pressure applied at this point stimulates the circulation of qi and blood, transmitting vital information through the meridian to the face and to the oral cavity to relieve the toothache and local swelling. This follows the principle cited in the *"Indications of Four Main Points in Verse"* to instruct in the clinical practice of Chinese acupuncture: "Choose the Hegu point for treating diseases of the face and mouth."

Through the study of Traditional Chinese Medicine over thousands of years, clinicians have discovered the following truths.

(1) Many acupuncture points lie on the meridians passing through the hand. Massage, acupuncture or moxibustion can be applied to stimulate these points to cure diseases and relieve discomfort throughout the whole body.

(2) As a miniature representation of the body, the hand — through changes in skin color, creases and sensitive points — can reveal the condition of all the organs and tissues of the body. At the same time, stimulation applied at the sensitive points can cure diseases in their corresponding organs and tissues.

At present, we can put a clear definition on the hand acupuncture therapy. It may be defined as a physiotherapy to prevent and treat diseases and relieve suffering by applying physical stimulation through acupuncture or massage on acupuncture points and areas on the hand. Before applying the treatment, the pathogenic factors should be determined, and a thorough diagnosis of the disease should be made by analyzing the information provided by the hand and the general pathological problems in the body.

The basic theories of hand acupuncture therapy include:

(1) The theory of Ba Gua (eight trigrams) on the palm

(2) The Zangfu (internal organs) and Jingluo (meridians and collaterals) theories of Traditional Chinese Medicine

(3) Modern biological theory of holographic embryo.

Compared with other therapies, acupuncture is a widely accepted and convenient therapeutic method to stimulate acupuncture points and areas on the hand. Therefore, it is often used in clinical practice where the treatment is simply called "hand acupuncture therapy."

Hand acupuncture therapy involves both diagnostic and therapeutic procedures. In the diagnostic aspect, observing only the hand itself — called "observation diagnosis of the hand" or "hand diagnosis"— is a unique way to provide detailed physiological and pathological information about the whole body. In the therapeutic aspect, the theories of both Traditional Chinese Medicine and Western medicine can be consulted to select the appropriate therapeutic method to be administered in clinical practice.

Section 2　Origin and Development of Hand Acupuncture Therapy

In Traditional Chinese Medicine, hand acupuncture therapy is an important branch of traditional acupuncture, both having been applied in clinical practice since ancient times. The meridians and acupuncture points, including many points on the hand, were already being mentioned in *Miraculous Pivot,* one of the volumes of *The Yellow Emperor's Canon of Medicine*, an ancient Traditional Chinese Medicine classic. For example, the three hand yang meridians that originate from the tips of the fingers and travel through the arm to the head and face have common acupuncture points along those meridians. On the hand, those acupoints are Shangyang (LI 1), Hegu (LI 4), Yangxi (LI 5), Shaoze (SI 1), Houxi (SI 3), Guanchong (SJ 1), Zhongzhu (SJ 3), and so on. The terminals of the three hand yin meridians also are located in the hand, and the common points in the hand of those meridians are Yuji (LU 10), Shaoshang (LU 11), Shaochong (HT 5), Laogong (PC 8), Zhongchong (PC 9), and so on. In addition, many lesser meridians are scattered throughout the hand, with their points such as Baxie (EX-UE 9), Shixuan (EX-UE 11), and so on. These observations recorded by ancient pioneers reveal the early discovery of the relationship between acupuncture points (sensitive or reactive spots) and the internal organs as well as the therapeutic effect produced by stimulating those points. For example, bleeding therapy applied at Shaoshang point can cure a sore throat and aphonia; therapy applied at the Shixuan points in children can control seizures caused by high fever. Such useful applications — passed on for thousands of years — have proved effective in clinical practice up to and including the present.

The history of hand diagnosis can be traced back to the Zhou Dynasty (c. 11th century-256 BC) when it was called "palmistry." There are many accounts of observation diagnosis in *The Yellow Emperor's Canon of Medicine*. For example, the *Miraculous Pivot* mentions "to examine internal organs and make a diagnosis of diseases through observing the superficial phenomena of human body;" the *Classic of Difficult Diseases* mentions "to make a diagnosis of diseases by observing five colors (of the face)." These references indicate that observations of superficial manifestations of problems in the body can show which organ is injured, what illness has been contracted and how the disease might be treated. Therefore, hand diagnosis is a really valuable procedure to find and analyze a disease. In ancient times in particular, the ability to learn and practice the observation method for diagnosis of diseases was considered a supreme skill. Clinicians who could make a correct diagnosis by the observation method alone were considered "miracle-working doctors." These doctors included Bian Que (c. 5th century) and Hua Tuo (?-205). Following them, a group of famous specialists displayed remarkable talent for the palmistry in the successive dynasties: Wang Yun in the Eastern Han Dynasty (25-220), Yuan Tiangang in the Tang Dynasty (618-907), Chen Tuan in the Song Dynasty (960-1279), and Guo Shanfu in the Yuan Dynasty (1271-1368).

In modern times, hand acupuncture therapy has made considerable progress and improvement. On the basis of traditional Zangfu and Jingluo theories and the diagram of hand acupuncture points, the modern Chinese specialists designed a new hand diagnosis diagram. By modifying the original hand diagnosis diagram of Jiu Gong (nine divisions) and Ba Gua (eight trigrams), the new diagram shows qi, color and appearance of the hand and the status of Zangfu (internal organs). With advantages of objectivity and accuracy, the new hand diagnosis diagram designed by Bai Lu and Zhang Yansheng was highly rated by practitioners. The author considers the traditional hand diagnosis diagrams undoubtedly useful in the diagnosis of diseases, but the newly-designed diagrams also are very valuable in the diagnosis and prognosis of diseases. The author will discuss their essentials and clinical applications in Chapter 3 and Chapter 4 of this book.

In the past ten or so years, the application of "massage at reflecting areas on the palm" has become more popular in Western countries, particularly in Europe and the USA. According to the theory of nerve reflex, reflex areas corresponding to most organs of the whole body are located in the palm for the diagnosis and treatment of diseases, so it is also called "reflexology."

Following the progress of modern biology in the past 20 years, theoretical studies in hand acupuncture therapy have hastened development and accumulation of new knowledge in the field. In 1973, Zhang Yingqin announced that he had discovered a biological holographic phenomenon and established a holographic embryo therapy. He believed that all living organisms, as well as any of their parts, can be considered independent holographic embryos that may be as small as a cell or as big as the whole organism. According to his theory, the hand of human body is actually a holographic embryo, too. A specific holographic embryo of the hand can show the characteristics of any part of the body and provide information about the whole body. Now, hand acupuncture therapy with a history over thousands years could be interpreted through the scientific holographic embryo theory. Therefore, rapid progress can be expected in the future study of hand acupuncture therapy under the guidance of evolving modern scientific theories.

CHAPTER 2
THEORIES OF HAND ACUPUNCTURE THERAPY

Section 1　Hand and Theory of Jiu Gong and Ba Gua

I.　What is Ba Gua?

The specific term, Ba Gua, first appeared in a unique ancient Chinese book, *Zhou Yi (The Book of Changes)*. Ba Gua are eight basic figures (trigrams) composed of two symbols, (--) Yinyao and (-) Yangyao, and their names are Qian Gua (☰), Kun Gua (☷), Zhen Gua (☳), Xun Gua (☴), Kan Gua (☵), Li Gua (☲), Gen Gua (☶), and Dui Gua (☱). In this book, Ba Gua are arranged to represent and explain eight natural phenomena. The Qian, Kun, Zhen, Xun, Kan, Li, Gen and Dui Gua represent the heaven, earth, thunder, wind, water, fire, mountain, and lake respectively. On the bases of the eight trigrams mentioned above, more trigrams (double trigrams) can be composed of Yinyao and Yangyao to represent all things in the universe to explain their change and development.

Ba Gua can also be used to represent and explain the human body. As the ruling heaven, Qian Gua corresponds to the head and brain; as earth, Kun Gua corresponds to the stomach, spleen and colon; as thunder, Zhen Gua corresponds to the liver and gallbladder; as wind, Xun Gua corresponds to the liver; as water, Kun Gua corresponds to the kidney; as fire, Li Gua corresponds to the heart; as mountain, Gen Gua corresponds to the spleen and small intestine; and as lake, Dui Gua corresponds to the lung.

II. Invention of Jiu Gong and Ba Gua

In ancient times, our ancestors divided the sky into nine fields, the earth into nine states and the human body into nine compartments with their particular numerals and fixed locations. As mentioned in an ancient book, *Luoshu*, "the numerals 2 and 4 are on both shoulders, 6 and 8 are at both feet, 3 is on the left side and 7 on the right, 9 is on the top and 1 at the bottom, and 5 is in the center." In the Han Dynasty (206 BC-AD 220), Zheng Xuan combined Jiu Gong and Ba Gua together to establish a Jiu Gong and Ba Gua theory. The numerals of Jiu Gong and locations of Ba Gua were defined in the Fig. 1.

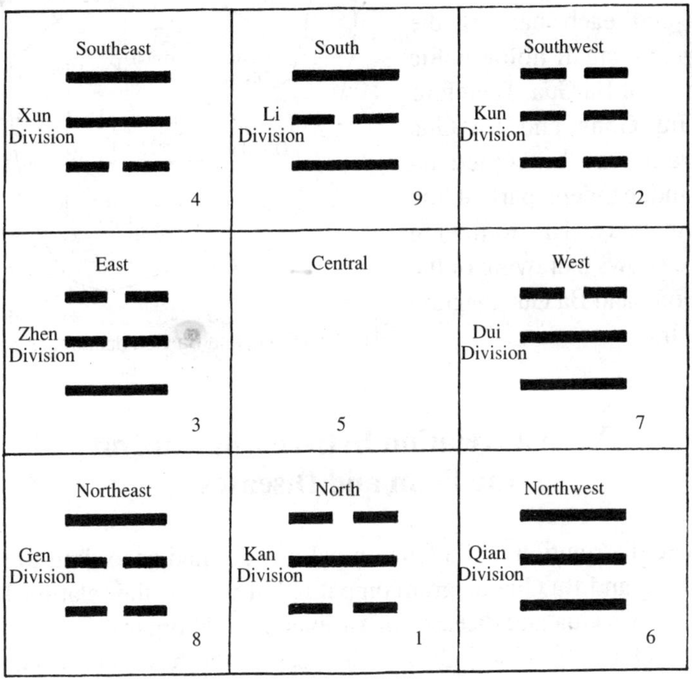

Fig. 1 Diagram to show orientation of Jiu Gong and Ba Gua

III. Distribution of Jiu Gong and Ba Gua on the Palm

This is actually a miniature holographic diagram of the universe. Ba Gua (eight trigrams) is a holographic diagram of the large universe and each trigram is a holographic diagram of a small universe, hence 64 trigrams (eight single trigrams plus 56 double trigrams with one trigram overlapped on the top of another one) make a complete Ba Gua system to indicate all things in the universe. In the same rules, the human body as a whole is a large holographic diagram of Ba Gua and each part of the body is a small holographic diagram of Ba Gua. Therefore, the Jiu Gong and Ba Gua diagram may be copied on any independent part of the human body. The following figure shows a drawing of the Jiu Gong and Ba Gua diagram on palm.

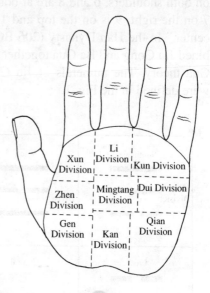

Fig. 2 Jiu Gong and Ba Gua diagram on palm

IV. Correlation Between Ba Gua on the Palm and Diseases

The distribution of Ba Gua on palm is defined according to the Jiu Gong and Ba Gua diagram on palm, but what is the relationship between Ba Gua and diseases of various internal organs?

1. Qian ($\equiv$) Gua indicates diseases of the head, chest, bones and colon, chronic diseases, constipation, and obstructive diseases.

2. Kun ($\equiv\equiv$) Gua indicates diseases of the abdomen, stomach,

intestine and skin, stagnation of food, edema due to excessive dampness, weakness of muscles, and tiredness.

3. Zhen (☳) Gua indciates diseases of the liver, enlargement of liver, flaming up of liver fire, psychosis, mania, epilepsy, convulsion, gynecological diseases, sore throat, and cough.

4. Xun (☴) Gua indicates the common cold, stroke, diseases of biliary tract, muscle spasms, and depression.

5. Kan (☵) Gua indciates diseases of the kidney, bladder and urinary system; diarrhea due to deficiency of kidney, diabetes mellitus, diseases of waist and back.

6. Li (☲) Gua: It indicates diseases of the heart and eye, febrile diseases, hyperplasia of the mammary gland, hypertrophy of the prostate gland.

7. Gen (☶) Gua indicates diseases of the stomach, anorexia, arthralgia, blood stasis in blood vessels, and lithiasis.

8. Dui (☱) Gua indicates diseases of the lung and chest, cough, shortness of breath, and bronchitis.

In brief, the location and severity of diseases can be determined by observing the divisions of Ba Gua on the palm and analyzing the relationship between Ba Gua and the diseases, no matter where they are located in the body. In any case, the theory of Jiu Gong and Ba Gua is constructed on the basis of ancient ideology. Therefore, the theory is too sweeping to instruct study of the very complicated human body (as a miniature universe) or make diagnosis of various diseases. On the other hand, it continues to play an important role in clinical practice as a basic principle and useful method to follow the location of diseases.

Section 2   The Hand and the Theory of Zangfu and Jingluo

As mentioned in textbooks of Traditional Chinese Medicine, the diagnosis and treatment of various diseases can be carried out through acupuncture points on the hand because the hand is closely connected with the Zangfu (internal organs) and Jingluo (meridian and collaterals) of the whole body. The Jingluo system can adjust the circulation of qi and blood, keep a balance of yin and yang in Zangfu, connect different (upper versus lower and inner versus outer) parts of the human body, and transport qi and blood to nourish the whole body. Therefore, a study of the integral connection between the hand and the Jingluo system is very important for illuminating the theory of hand acupuncture therapy.

I. Links Between the Hand and the 12 Meridians

First, the Jingluo system is composed of meridians and collaterals. A meridian is a trunk, and a collateral is a branch of a meridian. The meridian system is composed of 12 regular meridians and eight extra meridians. The 12 regular meridians include three hand and three foot yin meridians and three hand and three foot yang meridians that connect directly to their corresponding Zangfu. The 12 regular meridians have their definite routes to travel with a fixed sequence of top-to-bottom connections for transporting qi and blood. At the same time, there are many acupuncture points distributed on all the regular meridians. In the *Miraculous Pivot*, the routes the 12 meridians travel are mentioned in detail. The hand Taiyin lung meridian, hand Shaoyin heart meridian and hand Jueyin pericardium meridian originate in their corresponding organs in the chest and travel to reach the tips of fingers. The hand Yangming large intestine meridian, hand Taiyang small intestine meridian and hand Shaoyang Sanjiao meridian originate in the tips of the fingers and travel through the lateral aspect of the arm to end in the face and head. Therefore, six out 12 regular meridians link their corresponding organs directly to the hand.

Secondly, the 12 regular meridians are end-to-end linked with each other. The three hand yin meridians travel from the chest to the tips of fingers to connect with three hand yang meridians. The three hand yang meridians travel from the tips of fingers to the face and head to meet the three foot yang meridians. The three foot yang meridians travel from the face and head to the tips of toes to link with three foot yin meridians. The three foot yin meridians travel from the tips of toes to the chest and abdomen to make an endless circuit for communication of yin and yang. The endless circuit of 12 regular meridians can ensure the circulation of qi and blood in the circuit and conduct an intimate cooperation among various tissues and organs in the body. Therefore — because all regular meridians are connected with each other in sequence — stimulation applied to the acupuncture points of a meridian not only can promote the circulation of qi and blood through the meridian itself but also can activate the circulation of qi and blood through other meridians to adjust activities and functions of the whole body.

Because a close connection exists between the hand and the 12 meridians, the location of a disease can be determined by a hand diagnosis, and the disease can be treated with hand acupuncture therapy.

II.   Links Between the Hand and the 12 Meridianal Muscles

The twelve meridianal muscles are connected with the 12 meridians and nourished by qi and blood in the meridians to control the movement of bones and muscles. Therefore, these muscles are also in an intimate correlation with the hand. Following the routes of the 12 meridians on the body surface, the 12 meridianal muscles travel underneath the skin, from the ends of the four limbs to the head and trunk, then assemble around the joints and bones. The three hand yang and three hand yin meridianal muscles originate from the tips of fingers, travel along with their corresponding meridians and stop at the medial or lateral side of the arm, but some of them enter the chest and abdomen. Therefore, stimulation applied to acupuncture points and areas on the hand can also produce a therapeutic effect through the linkage of meridianal muscles with their corresponding Zangfu.

III. Links Between the Hand and the 12 Meridianal Skin Regions

The twelve meridianal skin regions are the cutaneous portions of 12 meridians for the spread and supply of meridianal qi to the body surface. Any change of color, tone or other appearance of the skin of the hand can indicate a dysfunction in a corresponding region of the body and pathological lesions of the correlated Zangfu and Jingluo. Therefore, acupuncture, moxibustion or hot compression applied to the skin of the hand can cure a disease of the internal organs. The theory of meridianal skin regions further proves the close relationship between the hand and the meridian system.

Section 3   The Hand and the Holographic Embryo System for Local Acupuncture

I.   The Biological Holographic Principle and the Holographic Embryo

Before explaining the holographic phenomena, the concept of biological holographic principle and holographic embryo must first be grasped.

In 1973, Zhang Yingqing, a Chinese medical scholar, announced that he had discovered a group of holographic acupuncture points beside the second metacarpal bone. They are arranged in a sequence from the distal end of the bone to its proximal end to assume a miniature of the human body from the head to the foot. This group of "holographic acupuncture points along the second metacarpal bone" has a whole new significance, because the points are completely different from traditional acupuncture points on the meridians. After further study, Zhang found various groups of holographic acupuncture points along other long bones, similar to the points along the second metacarpal bone. Zhang expanded his study to the whole biological field and found that the metamorphic bud of the cactus is also a small holographic embryo, so it is possible to grow a new plant from a cutting from the mother plant. After the mitotic division of a fertilized human ovum and semi-preserved duplication of DNA to grow a new individual, the somatic cells of the human body retain a copy of identical genes of the fertilized ovum. Therefore, the somatic cells can also play a role in growing a new organism as the fertilized ovum and embryo does. After a series of studies on many kinds of animals and plants, Zhang claimed that the root, stem, flower, leaf and fruit of plants and the head, limb, organs and tissues of animals (including human beings) may be considered as holographic embryos in different developing stages to grow a new organism. Hence all these may be called "holographic embryo," too.

In brief, any anatomically and functionally independent part of a living organism may be considered as a holographic embryo. In multiple cellular organisms, the structure between a single cell and their whole body can be divided into different developing stages. The whole body of an organism is in the highest developmental stage and the fertilized ova and somatic cells are in the lowest development stage. They are at two extremes of development. The tissues, organs and systems of an organism are the structures between both extremes to form a complete developmental sequence. The basic idea of the holographic embryo principle was born from above-mentioned holographic phenomena of the biosphere and is the principle used to define the developing stage of different structures in a living body.

As a common biological rule, the holographic embryo theory reveals the existence of a universal connection between each independent part of an organism and its whole body. The connection also exists among different parts of an organism.

II. The Hand and the Human Holographic Embryo System for Local Acupuncture

According to the holographic embryo theory, the author divided the developmental course of an organism into four stages from a fertilized ovum to a mature individual:

(1) The fertilized ovum and somatic cells of an organism are in the lowest developing stage of the holographic embryo.

(2) The epithelial, connective, muscular and nervous tissues are in the lower developing stage.

(3) The organs, such as the skin, muscle, bone, eye, nose, tongue, face, hand, and foot are in the higher developing stage.

(4) The whole mature organism is in the highest developing stage.

The author believes that the holographic embryos of higher maturity bear higher similarity among them and share more biological characteristics in common. The ear, eye, nose, tongue, face and foot for local acupuncture (now widely adopted at home and abroad) are similar miniatures of the whole human body. Therefore, all of them may be jointly used to show the physiological and pathological disturbances of the body. At the same time, they can be used to apply local acupuncture. Because hand acupuncture therapy is no exception, we may bring all varieties of local acupuncture, including hand acupuncture, into a common therapy group, the holographic embryo system for local acupuncture.

In brief, as a miniature of the whole human body, the hand is a highly developed holographic embryo. The acupuncture points and areas on the hand not only can show the physiological and pathological disturbances of their corresponding parts in the body but also can serve as the targets to apply local acupuncture to treat diseases of the corresponding parts. Therefore, the practice of hand diagnosis and hand acupuncture therapy is based on solid scientific theory and clinical experience.

In this chapter, the theories of the hand acupuncture therapy have been discussed. The gradual progress and improvement of those theories and the clinical practice of hand acupuncture is of course closely related to the development of human society and the advancement of science. The holographic integration theory of the universe was derived from the theory of Jiu Gong and Ba Gua in *The Book of Changes*. According to this theory, the human body is regarded as a miniature of the universe and at the same time, the whole human body or any independent part of the body is considered as a holographic diagram of Ba Gua. The theory is used to broadly explaing the doctrine of the inevitable connection between the hand and the whole body of human beings. Following further development of the theory of Zangfu and Jingluo and the accumulation of rich clinical experience in the Qin and Han Dynasties, it was established that the communication between the hand and whole body was carried out through the meridianal system. The new microscopic discovery about the close connection of hand and body has increased markedly the indications of hand acupuncture in clinical practice up to the present time. In the past 20 years, the traditional ear, nose, eye, face, hand and foot acupuncture therapies all have been incorporated into the holographic embryo system for local acupuncture. Following the establishment of holographic embryo theory and biological holographic principle, a modern biological significance has been attached to these traditional therapies. Since then, the theory of hand acupuncture therapy has become more and more scientific and systematic to guide the clinical practice of the therapy.

CHAPTER 3
LOCATION, NAME AND INDICATIONS OF HAND ACUPUNCTURE POINTS

Section 1 Hand Acupuncture Points of the Three Hand Yin and Three Hand Yang Meridians

Among the 12 regular meridians, those that pass through the hand are: The hand Taiyin lung, hand Shaoyin heart, hand Jueyin pericardium, hand Taiyang small intestine, hand Yangming large intestine, and hand Shaoyang Sanjiao meridians. The acupuncture points on those meridians are listed as follows (see Fig. 3 and Fig. 4).

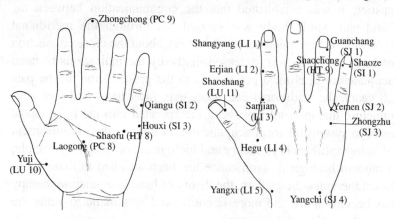

Fig. 3 Points of three Yin meridians on palm

Fig. 4 Points of three Yang meridians on dorsum of hand

16

1. Yuji (LU 10)

Location: A depression proximal to the first metacarpopharlangeal joint, on the radial side of the midpoint of the first metacarpal bone, at the junction of the skin on the back of the hand and skin of the palm.

Indications: Febrile diseases, sore throat, cough with much sputum, asthma and chest distress.

2. Shaoshang (LU 11)

Location: On the radial side of the distal segment of thumb, 0.1 cun from the fingernail.

Indications: Nasal bleeding, sore throat, severe stroke, and cough with shortness of breath.

3. Shangyang (LI 1)

Location: On the radial side of the distal segment of index finger, 0.1 cun from the corner of fingernail.

Indications: Tinnitus, deafness, dryness in the mouth, swelling of the cheek, blindness due to optic atrophy, diseases of the head, face and throat, and febrile diseases.

4. Erjian (LI 2)

Location: Distal to the second metacarpophalangeal joint, in a depression on the radial side of the joint when making a loose fist

Indications: Toothache, sore throat, nasal bleeding, blurred vision and febrile diseases.

5. Sanjian (LI 3)

Location: Proximal to the second metacarpophalangeal joint, in a depression on the radial side of the joint when making a loose fist.

Indications: Dental caries, eye pain, febrile diseases and sore throat.

6. Hegu (LI 4)

Location: On the dorsum of the hand, between the first and second metacarpal bones, on the radial side of the midpoint of second metacarpal bone.

Indications: Headache, facial paralysis, toothache, swelling of the cheeks, facial muscle spasms, nasal obstruction or runny nose, febrile disease and hand paralysis.

7. Yangxi (LI 5)

Location: At the radial end of the wrist crease, in a depression between the tendons of the short and long extensor muscles of the thumb when it is tilting up.

Indications: Redness, swelling and pain in the eyes and speech disorders.

8. Shaofu (HT 8)

Location: In the palm, between the fourth and fifth metacarpal bones, at point where the tip of little finger touches the palm when making a fist.

Indications: Hot feeling in the central portion of the palm, difficult urination, malaria, swelling and pain of the tongue, and pain of the arm and elbow.

9. Shaochong (HT 9)

Location: On the radial side of the distal segment of little finger, 0.1 cun from the corner of fingernail.

Indications: Febrile diseases with despondence, heart pain and shortness of breath.

10. Shaoze (SI 1)

Location: On the ulnar side of the distal segment of little finger, 0.1 cun from the corner of nail.

Indications: Sore throat, stroke, insufficient milk-secretion, nebula, febrile diseases, and loss of consciousness.

11. Qiangu (SI 2)

Location: At the junction of the skin on the back of the hand and skin of the palm along the ulnar border of hand, at the ulnar end of the crease of fifth metacarpophalangeal joint when making a loose fist.

Indications: Tinnitus, febrile diseases without sweat, dizziness and distension of head, mental instability.

12. Houxi (SI 3)

Location: At the junction of the skin on the back of the hand and skin of the palm along the ulnar border of hand, at the ulnar end of the distal palmar line (heaven line [heart line]), and proximal to the fifth metacarpophalangeal joint when making a hollow fist.

Indications: Headache with a stiff neck, stiffness of the neck, occipital headache, soreness in arms and shoulders, elbow pain, deafness and tinnitus, inflammation of the meatus of the outer ear, epilepsy and madness.

13. Wangu (SI 4)

Location: On the ulnar border of hand, in a depression between the proximal end of fifth metacarpal bone and the hamate bone, at the junction of the skin on the back of the hand and skin of the palm.

Indications: Jaundice, lockjaw, swelling of the cheeks, loss of consciousness, and febrile diseases.

14. Laogong (PC 8)

Location: At the center of palm, between the second and third metacarpal bones, but closer to the latter, at the point where the middle finger touches the palm when making a fist.

Indications: Febrile diseases, vomiting, nose bleeds, hiccups, epilepsy and madness, and loss of consciousness.

15. Zhongchong (PC 9)

Location: At the tip of middle finger.

Indications: Heart pain with despondence, febrile diseases without sweat, severe stroke, and loss of consciousness.

16. Guanchong (SJ 1)

Location: On the ulnar side of the distal segment of fourth finger, 0.1 cun from the corner of fingernail.

Indications: Sore throat, twisted tongue, heart pain with despondence and chest constriction.

17. Yemen (SJ 2)

Location: On the dorsum of hand, proximal to the border of the web between the fourth and fifth fingers, at the junction of the skin on the back of the hand and skin of the palm.

Indications: Vertigo, redness of the eyes, deafness and tinnitus, sore throat, and febrile diseases.

18. Zhongzhu (SJ 3)

Location: On the dorsum of hand, proximal to the fourth meta-carpophalangeal joint, in a depression between the fourth and fifth metacarpal bones.

Indications: Febrile diseases without sweat, headache, nebula and deafness.

19. Yangchi (SJ 4)

Location: At the midpoint of the dorsal crease of the wrist, in a depression on the ulnar side of the tendon of the extensor muscle of fingers.

Indications: Diabetes mellitus with dryness of the mouth, sore throat, febrile diseases, and pain in the hands and wrists.

Section 2 Specific and Extra Meridianal Hand Acupuncture Points

Specific and extra meridianal acupuncture points can produce a special therapeutic effect. Having been adopted into clinical practice for a long time, most of these points have proved particularly effective in treating a variety of diseases. They are mentioned as follows (see Fig. 5 and Fig. 6).

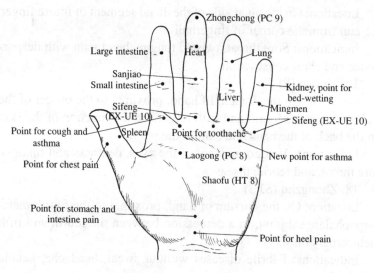

Fig. 5 Points for hand acupuncture (palm)

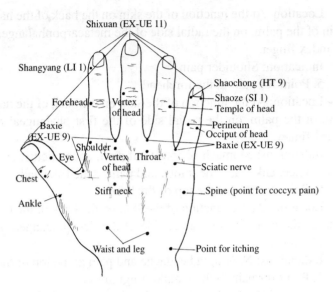

Shixuan (EX-UE 11)

Shangyang (LI 1)

Forehead — Vertex of head

Baxie (EX-UE 9)

Shoulder

Eye — Vertex of head — Throat

Chest

Stiff neck

Ankle

Waist and leg

Shaochong (HT 9)

Shaoze (SI 1)
Temple of head

Perineum
Occiput of head
Baxie (EX-UE 9)

Sciatic nerve

Spine (point for coccyx pain)

Point for itching

Fig. 6 Points for hand acupuncture (dorsum of hand)

1. Point for pain of medial malleolus

Location: At the junction of the skin on the back of the hand and skin of the palm, on the radial side of the metacarpophalangeal joint of thumb.

Indication: Ankle pain.

2. Point for chest pain

Location: At the junction of the skin on the back of the hand and skin of the palm, on the radial side of the phalangeal joint of thumb.

Indications: Chest pain, vomiting and diarrhea.

3. Point for eye pain

Location: At the junction of the skin on the back of the hand and skin of the palm, on the ulnar side of the phalangeal joint of the thumb.

Indication: Eye pain.

4. Point for shoulder pain

Location: At the junction of the skin on the back of the hand and skin of the palm, on the radial side of the metacarpophalangeal joint of index finger.

Indication: Shoulder pain.

5. Point for pain in the forehead

Location: At the junction of the skin on the back of the hand and skin of the palm, on the radial side of the first phalangeal joint of index finger.

Indications: Stomach or intestinal pain, appendicitis, arthralgia of the knee, ankle and toe joints, and pain in the forehead.

6. Point for pain at the top of the head

Location: At the junction of the skin on the back of the hand and skin of the palm, on the radial side of the first phalangeal joint of middle finger.

Indications: Neuralgia headache and pain at the top of the head.

7. Point for pain in the temple (migraine)

Location: At the junction of the skin on the back of the hand and skin of the palm, on the radial side of the first phalangeal joint of the ring finger.

Indications: Migraine, chest and side pain, pain of the liver or gallbladder, intercostal neuralgia, and pain of the spleen.

8. Point for pain of the perineum

Location: At the junction of the skin on the back of the hand and skin of the palm, on the radial side of the first phalangeal joint of little finger.

Indication: Pain in the perineum.

9. Point for pain in the back of the head

Location: At the junction of the skin on the back of the hand and skin of the palm, the ulnar side of the first phalangeal joint of little finger.

Indications: Pain in the back of the head and tonsillitis.

10. Point for back pain

Location: At the junction of the skin on the back of the hand and skin of the palm, on the ulnar side of the metacarpophalangeal joint of the little finger.

Indications: Acute sprain of the interspinal ligament and prolapse of an intervertebral disc.

11. Point for pain in the sciatic nerve (sciatica)

Location: Between the fourth and fifth metacarpophalangeal joints, closer to the former joint.

Indications: Sciatica and pain in the hip and buttocks.

12. Point for pain in the throat and tooth ache

Location: Between the third and fourth metacarpophalangeal joints, closer to the former joint.

Indications: Acute tonsillitis, sore throat and trigeminal neuralgia.

13. Point for neck pain

Location: Between the second and third metacarpophalangeal joints, closer to the former joint.

Indications: Stiff neck and neck sprain.

14. Point for lumbago

Location: On the radial side of the second extensor digitorum, on the ulnar side of the fourth extensor digitorum, and 1.5 cun proximal to the dorsal wrist crease.

Indications: Lumbago and sprain of the lower back.

15. Point for pain of stomach and intestine

Location: At the midpoint between Laogong (PC 8) and Daling (PC 7) points.

Indications: Chronic gastritis, peptic ulcer and indigestion.

16. Point for asthma and cough

Location: In the palm, on the ulnar side of the metacarpophalangeal joint of index finger.

Indications: Bronchitis, cough and asthma.

17. Point for bed-wetting and frequent urination

Location: On the palmar side of the little finger, at the midpoint of its second phalangeal crease .

Indications: Bed-wetting and frequent urination.

18. Point for pain in the heel

Location: At the midpoint between the point for stomach and intestine pain and Daling (PC 7) point.

Indication: Pain in the heel.

19. Point to raise blood pressure

Location: At the midpoint of the dorsal wrist crease.

Indication: For low blood pressure from any cause.

20. Point for hiccups

Location: On the dorsum of middle finger, at the midpoint of its second phalangeal crease.

Indication: Hiccups.

21. Point for high fever

Location: On the dorsum of hand, on the web between index and middle finger.

Indications: High fever and diseases of the eyes.

22. Point for diarrhea

Location: On the dorsum of the hand, 1 cun proximal to the junction between the third and fourth metacarpophalangeal joint.

Indication: Diarrhea.

23. Point for malaria

Location: At the junction of the first metacarpal bone and wrist joint, on the radial border of the thenar prominence.

Indication: Malaria.

24. Point of tonsillitis

Location: In the palm, at the midpoint of the ulnar border of first metacarpal bone.

Indications: Tonsillitis and sore throat.

25. Point for emergency treatment

Location: About 0.2 cun from the border of nail of the middle finger.

Indication: Coma.

26. Point to control epilepsy

Location: At the middle point of the border between the thenar and hypothenar prominence.

Indication: Epilepsy and fainting.

27. Point of the spleen

Location: On the palmar side of thumb, at the midpoint of its interphalangeal crease.

Indications: Diseases of spleen and stomach, and tumors.

28. Point of the small intestine

Location: On the palmar side of index finger, at the midpoint of the crease between its first and second phalangeal bone.

Indication: Diseases of small intestine.

29. Point of the large intestine

Location: On the palmar side of the index finger, at the midpoint of the crease between its second and third phalangeal bone.

Indication: Diseases of the large intestine.

30. Point of Sanjiao

Location: On the palmar side of middle finger, at the midpoint of the crease between its first and second phalangeal bone.

Indications: Diseases in chest, abdomen and pelvic cavity.

31. Point of the heart

Location: On the palmar side of the middle finger, at the midpoint of the crease between its second and third phalangeal bone.

Indication: Diseases of the heart and blood vessels.

32. Point of the liver

Location: On the palmar side of ring finger, at the midpoint of the crease between its first and second phalangeal bone.

Indication: Diseases of the liver and gallbladder.

33. Point of the lung

Location: On the palmar side of ring finger, at the midpoint of the crease between its second and third phalangeal bone.

Indication: Diseases of the respiratory system.

34. Point of Mingmen (life gate)

Location: On the palmar side of the little finger, at the midpoint of the crease between its first and second phalangeal bone.

Indication: Diseases of reproductive system.

35. Point of the kidney (night urination)

Location: On the palmar side of little finger, at the midpoint of the crease between its first and second phalangeal bone.

Indication: Diseases of kidney.

36. Dagukong (EX-UE 5)

Location: On the dorsal side of thumb, at the midpoint of its interphalangeal joint.

Indications: Diseases of the eyes, stomach ache and vomiting.

37. Xiaogukong (EX-UE 6)

Location: On the dorsal side of little finger, at the midpoint of its proximal interphalangeal joint.

Indications: Only for moxibustion to treat febrile diseases and diseases of eyes.

38. Yaotongdian (EX-UE 7)

Location: There are two points on the dorsum of each hand, between either the second and third or the fourth and fifth metacarpal bone, at the midpoint between the wrist crease and metacarpophalangeal joint.

Indications: Lumbago and hiccups.

39. Wailaogong (EX-UE 8)

Location: On the dorsum of hand, between the second and third metacarpal bone, 0.5 cun proximal to the metacarpophalangeal joint.

Indications: Stomach ache and abdominal pain.

40. Baxie (EX-UE 9)

Location: There are four points on the dorsal side of each hollow fist, on the junction between the skin on the back of the hand and skin of the palm just proximal to the border of all webs between the five fingers.

Indications: Febrile diseases and pain.

41. Sifeng (EX-UE 10)

Location: There are four points on the palmar side of the second to fifth fingers of each hand, at the midpoint of their proximal interphalangeal creases.

Indication: For pricking acupuncture to treat infantile malnutrition due to indigestion.

42. Shixuan (EX-UE 11)

Location: There is a point at each tip of the 10 fingers, 0.1 cun away from the free edge of nail.

Indications: Febrile diseases, hypertension and revival of patients in critical condition.

Section 3 Points and Areas of Hand Holographic Embryo System for Local Acupuncture

In recent years, several schools of acupuncture in the holographic embryo system have been established with different views. However, the opinions of the different schools can be organized into three groups:

In the first group, the traditional diagram of Ba Gua for hand diagnosis and treatment of diseases continues to be applied in clinical practice; in the second group, changes in lines on the palm are taken into account to diagnose and treat diseases; and in the third group, a combination of the "palm massage" diagram used in Western countries and the "hand diagnosis diagram" of Zhang Yansheng used at China is applied in clinical practice to make diagnosis according to qi, color and appearance of hand.

On the basis of personal experience and study, the author thinks that the last group is the most reasonable and scientific in its clinical practice and theoretical foundations. After rectifying and modifying the progress achieved by the specialists in the third group, the author has organized the hand holographic embryo system for local acupuncture as follows:

First of all, two basic lines should be defined. The first one on the palm is a line to connect the center of the base of middle finger and the midpoint of the wrist crease. It is used to represent the anterior midline of the body and the vertical axis in the body. The second line is drawn along the extensor tendon of the middle finger on the back of the hand to represent the posterior midline of human body. Following the first line from its distal end to the proximal end, the corresponding areas of head, nose, mouth, esophagus, stomach, kidney, reproductive organs and perineum are arranged in sequence.

Secondly, most people have four basic lines on their palms that are very useful in defining corresponding divisions of the internal organs. The distal horizontal line is called heaven or emotion line [heart line] and the proximal half-oblique one traveling along the medial border of thenar prominence is called earth, life or health line [life line]. The middle oblique one traveling downward from the left border to the right side (always watching the left hand as a rule) of the palm is called human being or career line [head line] and the vertical one as the midline of palm is called Yuzhu (jade post) or intelligence line [fate line].

In general, the divisions on the palm of hand represent the internal organs inside the human body and organs on the frontal wall of body; and the divisions on the dorsum of hand represent the organs on the back of the head, upper and lower back, and spine. The divisions on both sides of the hand are mentioned as follows (see Figs. 7-11).

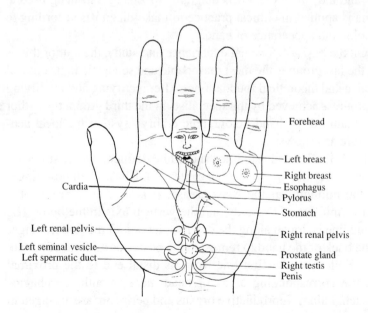

Fig. 7

1. Head area

Location: Around the palmar crease at the base of middle finger.

Indications: Diseases of the top of the head, forehead and both temples (Taiyang point).

2. Nose area

Location: On the vertical midline of the head area and just below the forehead.

Indications: Diseases of the nasal septum or nasal cavity.

3. Eye area

Location: Below the head area, beside the nose area and not beyond the interosseous spaces on both sides of the third metacarpal bone.

Indications: Disorder of visual acuity and diseases of the eyelids, fundus [back of the eye], cornea and iris.

4. Cheek area

Location: Below the eye area, beside the nose area and above the mouth area.

Indication: Diseases of cheek.

5. Mouth area

Location: Below the nose area and around the intersection of the vertical palmar midline and the heaven line [heart line].

Indications: Diseases of the teeth, cheeks, tongue, oral mucosa and throat.

6. Esophagus area

Location: Below the mouth area, on the vertical palmar midline between the heaven line [heart line] and the human being line [head line] with its proximal end as the cardia area.

Indications: Diseases of the esophagus, cardia, neck, thyroid and parathyroid gland.

7. Stomach area

Location: Around the midpoint of the vertical palmar midline.

Indications: Diseases of stomach, cardia, pylorus and duodenum.

8. Kidney area

Location: Next to the vertical palmar midline, on both sides of the midpoint between the center of the stomach area and the midpoint of the wrist crease.

Indications: Diseases of renal pelvis, adrenal gland and renal tubules.

9. Area of reproductive organs

Location: Around the midpoint between the center of the kidney area and the midpoint of the wrist crease.

In males, the upper portion of this area on both sides represents the seminal vesicle and spermatic duct; the lower portion of the area represents the testis and ependidymis; and the central portion represents the prostate gland.

In females the right hand is observed. The upper portion represents the appendage (ovary and oviduct); the central portion represents the uterus; and the lower portion represents the uterine cervix and vagina respectively (see Fig. 9).

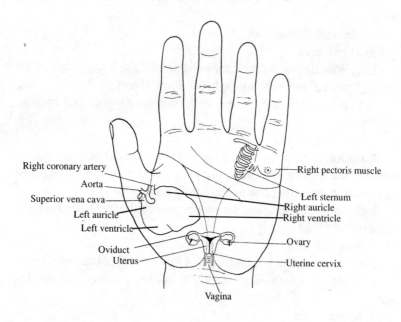

Fig.9

Indications: Diseases of prostate gland, testis, ependidymis, seminal vesicle, and spermatic duct in male; and diseases of uterus, vagina, oviduct and ovary in female.

10. Trachea area

Location: A vertical rectangular area from the web between the ring and little finger to the heaven line [heart line]. Diseases of lung and trachea are shown in this area (see Fig. 8).

Indication: Diseases of trachea.

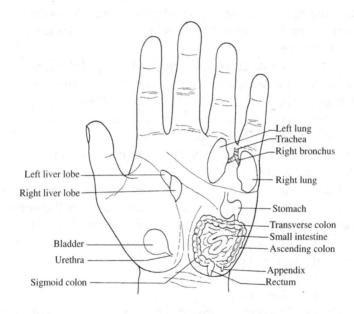

Fig. 8

11. Area of left chest and lung

Location: On the left side of the trachea area.

Indications: Diseases of the left chest, bronchus, lung, pleura, ribs, breast and upper back.

12. Area of right chest and lung

Location: The midline of this area is coincides with the upper part of the fourth metacarpal bone distal to the heaven line [heart line] to represent the vertical midline of the right chest wall.

Indications: Diseases of the right chest, bronchus, lung, pleura, ribs, breast and upper back.

13. Lower back and waist area

Location: The intersection of the vertical midline of the trachea area and the heaven line [heart line] is Yaoyan (EX-B 7) point, on both sides of the point lies a horizontal area over the heaven line [heart line] (from the interosseous space between the middle and ring finger to the ulnar border of palm) to represent both sides of the waist.

Indications: Diseases of lumbar spinal column and waist.

14. Liver area

Location: A triangular area surrounded by the interosseous space between the index and middle finger, human being line [head line] and earth line [life line] as its three edges. The medial portion of this area represents the small left lobe and the lateral portion represents the large right lobe of the liver.

Indications: Diseases of liver, enlargement of liver and hepatitis.

15. Spleen area

Location: An area between the heaven line [heart line] and the human being line [head line] with its center situated at the intersection of a horizontal line passing through the center of the liver area and a vertical line drawn along the interosseous space between the metacarpal bones of the middle and ring finger.

Indication: Diseases of spleen.

16. Gallbladder area

Location: The center of this area is at the intersection of a horizontal line passing through the lower (proximal) angle of liver area (on the earth line [life line]) and a vertical line drawn through the center of trachea area. It is lower than (proximal to) the spleen area.

Indications: Diseases of gallbladder and biliary ducts.

17. Areas of the upper, middle and lower abdomen

Location: The center of the upper abdomen area is at the intersection of a tangential line of the human being [head line] and a vertical line drawn through the trachea area. The vertical midline of the hypothenar prominence is divided into three segments to divide the abdomen into the upper, middle and lower divisions (see Fig. 8).

Indications: Diseases in the organs of the abdomen such as the pancreas, peritoneal membrane, small intestine, appendix, stomach, and ascending, transverse and descending colon.

A unique characteristic of the right half of the palm is that it is "headless and tailless" (that is, it includes only the trunk of human body) to represent the organs between the neck and perineum. The corresponding areas of internal organs on the left half of the palm are mentioned as follows. First of all, the palmar surface of the proximal segment of the index finger is divided into three equal vertical portions.

18. Area for dreaminess

Location: In the left one-third of the proximal segment of index finger.

Indications: Insomnia and dreaminess.

19. Area for insomnia

Location: In the right one-third of the proximal segment of index finger.

Indications: Insomnia, sleepiness and nervous status.

20. Area for hypertension

Location: In the left one-third of the proximal segment of middle finger.

Indication: Hypertension.

21. Area for hypotension

Location: In the right one-third of the proximal segment of middle finger.

Indication: Hypotension.

22. Area for dizziness

Location: In the middle one-third of the proximal segment of middle finger.

Indications: Dizziness, Co poisoning and fainting.

23. Area for fatigue

Location: In a square area left to the intersection of the heaven line [heart line] and the interosseous space between the metacarpal bones of index and middle finger.

Indications: Annoyance, anger, decrease of body strength and poor mental concentration.

24. Area for poor blood supply

Location: In a depression on the right border of thenar prominence with the palm.

Indications: Anemia, poor blood supply to heart and angina pectoris.

25. Anus area

Location: In the prominent area around the tip of thumb, which is divided into the lateral, anterior, medial and posterior quarters to represent the left, front, right and rear parts of the anus.

Indications: Hemorrhoids, anal fissure and other diseases of the anus.

26. Rectum area

Location: In the prominent area from the tip of the thumb to the center of its finger pad. The vertical midline of this area divides it into lateral and medial sides to represent the left and right sides of rectum respectively.

Indications: Diseases of rectum, anus and sigmoid colon.

27. Area for deficiency of qi

Location: Distal to the heart area, on the junction of the skin on the back of the hand and skin of the palm over the medial surface of the proximal segment of thumb.

Indication: Diseases with deficiency of vital energy.

28. Heart area

Location: The thenar prominence is divided into two vertical portions with the medial one bigger than the lateral one to represent the right and left heart (both ventricle and auricle) respectively.

Indications: Diseases of heart and aorta.

29. Area for edema

Location: The lateral one-half of the thenar prominence is divided into three equal transverse portions and the upper one-third represents the left heart and the middle one-third is the area for edema.

Indication: Edema.

30. Area for rheumatism

Location: In the lower one-third of the lateral one-half of the thenar prominence.

Indications: Rheumatism, catching cold and common cold of the wind-cold type.

31. Bladder area

Location: The area is around the intersection of the interosseous space between the metacarpal bones of the index and middle finger and the midline of the thenar prominence, and it is below the heart area. The urethra area is below this area, on the wrist crease.

Indications: Diseases of urinary system, including urinary bladder, urethra and so on.

32. Skin area

Location: Directly below the area for hypertension, at the intersection of its midline and the right border of the thenar prominence.

Indications: Allergic dermatitis, eczema, purpura, subcutaneous hemorrhage, and anemia.

33. Area of the left shoulder and arm

Location: In an area of the palm left to a vertical line drawn from the left end of the basal crease of index finger to the human being line [head line].

Indications: Diseases of left shoulder and arm.

34. Area of the right shoulder and arm

Location: In the area of the palm right to a vertical line drawn from the right end of the basal crease of little finger to the heaven line [heart line].

Indications: Diseases of the right shoulder and arm.

35. Area of the left ear

Location: In the central area of the left surface of the proximal segment of middle finger.

Indications: Diseases of left outer meatus and eardrum, otitis media, and perforated eardrum.

36. Area of the right ear

Location: In the central area of the right surface of the proximal segment of middle finger.

Indications: Diseases of the right outer meatus and eardrum.

37. Area of back of the head (occipital bone)

Location: On the dorsal surface of thumb and around the phalangeal joint (see Fig. 10).

Indication: Occipital headache.

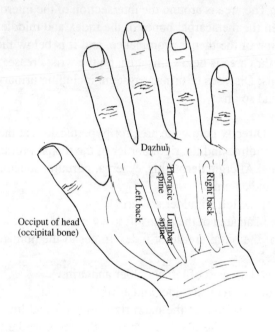

Fig. 10

38. Spine area

Location: Along the tendon of the extensor muscle of middle finger.

Indications: Diseases of cervical, thoracic and lumbar spine.

39. Cervical spine

Location: On the dorsal surface of hand, around the metacarpophalangeal joint of middle finger.

Indications: Diseases of cervical spine and both shoulders.

40. Thoracic spine area

Location: Below the area of the cervical spine, in an area over the upper three-fifths of the extensor tendon of the middle finger.

Indications: Diseases of the thoracic spine and upper back.

41. Lumbar area

Location: In an area over the lower two-fifths of the extensor tendon of the middle finger and above the dorsal wrist crease.

Indications: Diseases of waist, lumbar muscles and lumbar and sacral bones.

42. Back area

Location: The whole dorsum of hand represents the whole back of human body. The radial half of the dorsum of hand represents the left back; and its ulnar half represents the right back (see Fig. 11).

Indication: Diseases of the whole back.

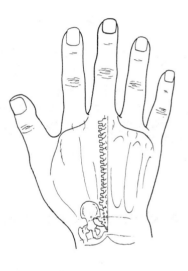

Fig. 11

CHAPTER 4
HAND OBSERVATION DIAGNOSIS

Observation diagnosis includes many diagnostic techniques such as observation of the shape of the fingers, shape of the hand, shape of the palm and patterns of palmar lines according to established principles of palmistry. Because of the limited range of this book, only two techniques used in hand diagnosis will be mentioned as follows:

Section 1 Observation Diagnosis on the Palm

I. Shape of the Palm

1. Round palm: A round palm is usually found in people with good health, abundant energy, indomitable will, and an extroverted and optimistic disposition. People with round palms seldom suffer from diseases caused by emotional disturbance or mental depression (see Fig. 12).

2. Square palm: A square palm is usually found in people with satisfactory health, a conscientious attitude toward work, an active lifestyle, but also with a stubborn disposition at times. They are susceptible to cardiovascular and cerebrovascular diseases in their later years (see Fig. 13).

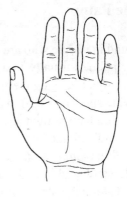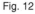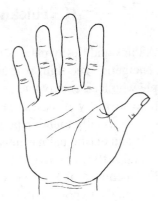

Fig. 12   Fig. 13

3. Spoon-shaped palm: A spoon-shaped palm with thick wrist and base of the fingers is usually found in people with an open-minded temperament, vigorous physical strength and self-confidence. If addicted to tobacco or alcohol, these people may be susceptible to lumbago and to being easily agitated and to early aging. (see Fig. 14).

4. Rectangular palm: A rectangular palm with thin palmar muscles is usually found in people who tend to be introverted, nervous, high-strung, sensitive and fearful. They are susceptible to poor memory and weak vitality due to poor health (see Fig. 15).

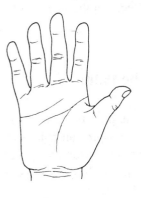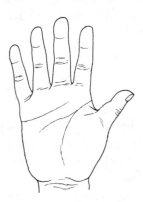

Fig. 14   Fig. 15

II. Thickness of the Palm

A thick and fleshy palm is usually found in people who are vital and energetic. The thin, soft and slender palm is usually found in people who lack energy and are physically weak, leaving them susceptible to many diseases. The palm with rigid and stiff palmar muscles is usually found in people with poor adaptability; therefore, the soft and elastic palmar muscles are an indication of strong physique and sufficient energy. The hard and thin palm is an indication of dysfunction of the digestive system. Lusterless skin and wasted muscles in the hypothenar prominence and along the ulnar border of the palm indicates deficiency of body fluid, usually caused by chronic diarrhea or dysentery.

III. Veins on the Palm

Engorged superficial veins on the back of the hand or in the crease of the phalangeal joint are usually found in people with intestinal blockage by hard feces. These people are susceptible to habitual constipation, hemorrhoids and venous aneurysm, but the engorged veins may gradually subside and disappear and the hemorrhage of hemorrhoids may stop after the hard feces in the intestine has been voided.

IV. Color of the Palm

The normal hand has a palm that is pink or light red in color, lustrous, moist, elastic and powerful in grasping an object. Once the palmar color turns darker or lighter for any reason other than weather changes or mental, physical or chemical influences — people will certainly show some deterioration in their health.

1. A pale palm indicates diseases of the lung. A dark palm

without luster indicates diseases of the kidney. A purplish palm indicates abnormal blood circulation. A bluish palm indicates intestinal problems. A greenish palm indicates anemia or disease of the stomach and spleen. The golden yellow palm indicates liver diseases. A crimson (deep red) palm indicates an excessiveness of heart fire. A pale or dark-blue palm indicates anemia, blood stasis, hypertension, hypotension, heart diseases, gout or an invisible hemorrhage — and the diagnosis of these diseases may be made without doubt if the abnormal color change can be found in the three main lines on the palm. Engorged veins on a dull palm indicate hemorrhoids. A red network of capillaries on the palm indicates a deficiency of vitamin C.

2. A palm with red or crimson patches on the thenar and hypothenar prominence — popularly known as "cinnabar palm" — indicates a past history of hepatitis, and so is also called a "liver palm." If the patches are dark purple in color, it indicates persistent hepatitis with most liver cells destroyed. Red patches may also appear on the palm of patients with a deficiency of vitamin C. The palm may be bright red in the color of patients with systemic lupus erythematosus.

3. The palm of cancer patients may be in a color of loess (yellowish brown) without luster. After chemotherapy, the color of the palm may turn to dark brown. A black palm and fingers indicates patients in critical condition in the late stages of disease due to the spread of toxic substances to the four limbs.

Section 2 Hand Diagnosis by Observation of Holographic Areas

Hand diagnosis is based on Traditional Chinese Medicine theory of observation diagnosis. Location of diseases for application of local acupuncture is determined by observing color and its changes in holographic areas of the hand. The naked eye looks to find any signs of excessive or deficient qi and blood in patients and to make a diagnosis and prognosis of diseases.

The advantages of this kind of diagnosis are as follows:

(1) Holographic area diagnosis is applied on the basis of both observation diagnosis theory of Traditional Chinese Medicine and holographic embryo theory.

(2) Diagnosis is simple, objective, regular, stable, and easy to learn and practice.

(3) In comparison with other observation diagnoses, it is more accurate.

(4) Diagnosis may be adopted as a supplemental method to other diagnostic measures of Traditional Chinese Medicine or Western medicine.

(5) Diagnosis can reveal latent diseases in time to prevent further their progress.

I. Analysis of the Five Colors and
Their Indications

Human skin color consists of five basic colors, blue, red, yellow, white and black, and these colors represent the five internal organs — liver, heart, spleen, lung and kidney. Lustrous and moist, the skin of the normal human hand is tinted with these five colors. The skin of the palm is redder, moister, and more delicate than the skin of the back of the hand. The above-mentioned normal appearance of the skin of the hand indicates that its owner is a person with sufficient essence, qi, blood and Jinye (body fluid), normal functions of Zang-fu and balanced yin and yang.

In patients, abnormal colors may appear, with one color in dominance over the others, either very dull and dark or extraordinarily bright. Ancient physicians divided abnormal colors into five basic categories of blue, red, yellow, white and black to indicate five groups of syndromes (patterns of disease). This is the so-called "indications of five colors."

1. Blue: Indicates a cold syndrome, pain syndrome, blood stasis syndrome or convulsion syndrome.

2. Red: Indicates a hot syndrome. A dark red color indicates an excessive hot syndrome and a light red color indicates a deficient hot syndrome.

3. Yellow: Indicates a deficient syndrome or damp syndrome.

4. White: Indicates a deficient syndrome or cold syndrome.

5. Black: Indicates a kidney-deficiency syndrome, cold syndrome, blood stagnation syndrome or phlegm retention syndrome.

The "indications of five colors" mentioned above is only a general principle of observation diagnosis, but indications may vary with changes in their location. Details of the "indications of colors" in different holographic areas are as follows:

1. White: In general, the color white indicates pain (ordinary pain), inflammation and stasis or deficiency of qi. If white is present in the whole kidney area, it indicates deficiency of kidney qi; and if present in the spleen and stomach area, it indicates deficiency of Zhongjiao (spleen and stomach) qi. White also indicates an internal cold syndrome.

2. Red: In general, the color red indicates the febrile or blood-congestion diseases, such as the hot syndrome, blood heat, blood congestion, stagnation of heat, and accumulation of heat.

3. Light red: In general, a light red color indicates impaired functions and poor vitality of Zangfu, including a disease with deficiency of superficial yang, disease in an early stage, chronic disease in a healing or recovery stage, and mild febrile disease.

4. Deep red: "A deep color always indicates an excessive syndrome" or heat syndrome. For example, in patients with the "liver palm," the skin over the thenar and hypothenar prominence is red with scattered dark red spots and patches because much heat has accumulated in the liver, known as "excessiveness of liver fire." In patients with habitual constipation over the years, a similar color change and red patches — caused by the accumulation of heat or

congestive inflammation in the abdomen, rather than in the liver — may also appear on the hypothenar prominence. In patients with dry cough and yellow sputum, the color red in the lung and bronchus areas indicates the presence of heat and inflammation in the lung. The appearance of a dark red color in the pharynx area indicates congestive pharyngitis with dryness and pain in the throat. If some white spots are scattered over the dark red pharynx area, the patients may suffer from congestive pyogenic disease, such as purulent tonsillitis.

5. Fresh red: Fresh red spots everywhere on the palm indicates the presence of bleeding in the corresponding organ, including spontaneous hemorrhaging and bleeding caused by operations and trauma. These red spots are different from the so-called Zhusha Zhi (minute hemangioma), although they look similar.

6. Dark red: A change of the fresh red color to a dark red color indicates that the hemorrhaging has stopped and the wound has begun to heal.

7. Purplish red: A purplish red color usually indicates blood stasis. It often appears in subcutaneous capillaries to show the presence of mild blood stasis, poor blood circulation or blood coagulated in a wound.

8. Deep coffee: A deep coffee color indicates that the disease is already cured, the operation incision or wound is almost healed up, and the black pigmented areas of the skin of a rather large size are present in the corresponding regions of the body.

9. Light coffee: A light coffee color usually appears deep beneath the skin of the palm to indicate a disease that has been cured a long time.

10. Blue: The symbolic color of the liver, blue indicates stagnation of the liver qi. Blue also indicates severe pain, because "pain is controlled and adjusted by the liver." The presence of some blue blood vessels underneath the skin indicates blood stasis in the blood vessels.

11. Bluish white: In general, bluish white indicates severe pain caused by stagnation of qi or an attack of bitter cold. In patients with

severe influenza, a bluish white color may appear on the lateral border of the thenar prominence.

12. Bluish purple: In general, bluish purple indicates a disease either in the early stage or in the recovery stage. Bluish purple color usually appears in the subcutaneous blood vessels of the palm to indicate a disturbance of blood quality, such as an increase of blood viscosity, contraction of capillaries, reduction of blood oxygen, abnormal contents of blood lipids and increase of acids in blood. Any disturbance of blood quality can cause dizziness and cold limbs as blood circulation slows to the terminal blood vessels.

The appearance of blue and purple subcutaneous blood vessels in the head area, area of occiput of head, area of cervical spine and the Dazhui (DU 14) area on the palm indicate poor blood circulation in the brain. If many blue or purple blood vessels are found here and there over the palm, patients may be susceptible to thrombosis or blood clotting in the brain, limbs and abdominal aorta due to the above-mentioned disturbance of blood quality and increase of blood coagulability.

13. Black (dark gray): A black or dark gray color on the palm and fingers (except the thumb) indicates an increase of blood lipids due to low metabolism. The waste products of metabolism are accumulated in the body to cause fatigue, lack of energy and reduction of mental power because the patient does not engage in enough physical exercise to consume their excessive nutrients.

14. Yellow: The palm of patients with liver and gallbladder diseases is usually yellow in color, particularly remarkable in patients with jaundice. In some infants, jaundice is hereditary in nature and caused by hemolysis due to incompatible blood types of their parents who have AB and O blood types respectively. Besides this serious hemolysis, a common infant jaundice is physiological in nature, but a severe infant jaundice still indicates a high susceptibility to diseases of liver, gallbladder and blood system. In general, a yellow palm indicates chronic diseases with a long clinical course. For example, yellow in the throat area indicates chronic pharyngitis. Yellow rough skin in the stomach area indicates

chronic gastritis. Mucosa of the stomach may be also thickened, if the yellow skin is thickened.

15. Dark colors (dark blue, dark gray and dark purple color): A variety of dark colors indicates the accumulation of too many foreign substances in the body.

16. Dark purple: Dark purple indicates diseases caused by deficiency of yin or functional disturbance in the body. Dark purple may also indicates organic diseases caused by a viral infection.

17. Dark blue and dark gray: In general, dark blue or dark gray indicates changes in the contents of the blood to cause skin problems or problems in deep subcutaneous regions due to poor blood supply. Examples would be subcutaneous hemorrhaging caused by reduction of blood platelets and increase of capillary fragility and skin diseases caused by an increase of acids in the blood.

18. Dark coffee: A dark coffee color usually appears in the area of cervical spine and the Dazhui (DU 14) area and on the back of the hand to indicate pain caused by an attack of wind or blockage to the circulation of qi and blood.

19. Pigmentation (age spots and areas of pigmentation): Areas of pigmentation may appear everywhere in the skin of patients with disturbance of endocrine system, dysfunction of internal organs and impairment of physique. Areas of pigmentation may also appear on the hand to indicate impaired functions of corresponding organs. With the exception of birthmarks, newborn babies seldom bear areas of pigmentation on their skin, but these areas may gradually appear and increase in number and size during aging because the metabolic burden on the liver gradually increases, decreasing its ability to detoxify. Areas of pigmentation may also appear in hand holographic areas following a continuous impairment of certain functions of the body. Pigment is evenly distributed in the skin all over the body in people with good health, vigorous metabolism and balanced functions among their organs, but pigmented spots and patches may appear in holographic areas of the hand following any physical impairment, attack of disease and decrease in the circulation of qi and blood.

II. Changes of Color and Appearance in Holographic Areas on the Hand and Differential Diagnosis of Syndromes

1. Head area

White around the crease of the metacarpophalangeal joint of middle finger indicates a headache. If the white color is located in the middle segment of the crease, it indicates a headache in the forehead and vortex of head; if white is located only in the left half of the crease, it indicates migraine on the left side of the head; and if only in the right half, it indicates migraine on the right side of the head. The presence of some blue, purplish red or bluish purple blood vessels underneath the white skin in youths indicates that the headache and dizziness is caused not only by stagnation of qi but also by blood stasis. The starvation of the brain due to decreased blood circulation in the head with poor blood supply to the brain may cause headache and dizziness.

2. Area for dizziness

The presence of a dark or light red, light or dark brown, or any dark color spreading upward from the bottom to the top of this whole area [See Chapter 3] indicates that the patient is susceptible to vertigo and dizziness caused by deficiency of qi or excessiveness of yin. The spread of a red color from this whole area to nearby areas for hypertension and for hypotension indicates dizziness with distending headache, usually caused by the upward rush of blood, hyperactivity of liver yang or "hepatic hypertension" (due to dysfunction of liver). A dark purple color in this area indicates dizziness due to poor blood supply and hypoxia of the brain. The presence of a yellowish brown callus-like papule (occasionally coffee or light yellow in color) on the palmar side of the proximal segment of middle finger indicates a persistent dizziness.

3. Area for hypertension

The presence of a red patch in this area with clear-cut margins indicates hypertension caused by an upward rush of blood or hyperactivity of liver yang, also known as "hepatic hypertension." A white color over the whole area indicates general hypertension; and a dark red or dark gray color in this area indicates renal hypertension.

4. Area for hypotension

A bright white color all over in this area indicates hypotension due to deficiency of qi and blood and poor supply of blood chiefly in women with dizziness, shortness of breath, anemia, hatred of cold, coolness and numbness of limbs.

5. Eye area (left and right eye)

A white color (sometimes slightly bulging) in this area indicates any inflammation in the eyes (trachoma, sty, and so on). A red color in this area indicates blood congestion of eyes. A gray, grayish blue or dark gray flat skin in this area indicates blurred vision, astigmitism, poor focusing of eyes. If some blue blood vessels can be seen beneath the skin in a gray or grayish color and the vessels extend to the head area, patients may suffer from impairment of vision caused by poor blood supply to the eye fundus or a restriction of cerebral blood circulation.

6. Nose area

A white color in this area indicates a temporary nasal infection or patients are suffering from an inflammation in the nasal cavity. The presence of a vertical dark callus-like rod along the midline of the area indicates chronic rhinitis. Depressed skin of this area in an uneven dark gray color, sometimes covered with fine lines, indicates atrophic rhinitis.

7. Mouth area

This is a holographic area of both the mouth and oral cavity to show their condition and diseases. A white color in this area indicates inflammation with pain, and a dark purple, dark gray or coffee color indicates chronic and relapsing pharyngitis.

8. Tooth and cheek areas

The presence of a white spot or small patch located in a certain part of this area indicates inflammation with pain in the corresponding tooth. The purity of the white matches the severity of the inflammation, so the whiter the skin in the tooth area looks, the more severe the inflammation afflicting the patient. The presence of a dark yellow or coffee-color bulging spot or patch in this area indicates chronic inflammation or caries (without severe pain) of the corresponding tooth, which may be filled or extracted.

9. Esophagus area

The white bulging skin in this area indicates edema of the esophagus. A red alternating with white color or pure red color in this area indicates esophagitis. An even pink patch with clear-cut radiating margins in the area indicates esophageal diverticulum. A red color indicates congestion or congestive inflammation of the esophagus. A blister-like papule in this area with red borders and an irregular shape indicates infiltrating inflammation or esophageal carcinoma.

10. Stomach area

The conjunction of the esophagus and stomach is the cardia, and the part of the stomach next to the kidney is the stomach fundus. White, shiny and depressed skin in the whole area indicates deficiency and coldness of the stomach. White, shiny and bulging skin over this area indicates edema of gastric mucosa. Yellow, rough and callus-like skin indicates thickening of gastric mucosa or chronic gastritis over a large area. Dark red color in this area indicates congestive inflammation or congestion of the gastric mucosa due to heat in the stomach. Patients may suffer from acid reflux, heartburn and bad breath. Dark depressed skin present in a local region of this area indicates atrophic gastritis. Bulging skin in a local region of this area with a dark or blackish brown color underneath the skin indicates chronic peptic stomcah ulcer.

11. Kidney area

White in this area indicates deficiency of kidney qi, and patients may suffer impotence and premature ejaculation of semen and — in both sexes — weakness in the lower back and the leg. A pink or light red color on the surface of the skin all over this area indicates deficiency of kidney yang, and patients may suffer from sexual disorders. A dark purple color or dark red color with some grayish tint all over this area indicates deficiency of kidney yin and a dysfunction of the kidney itself. Brownish yellow spots in the kidney area on one hand indicates chronic nephritis of the kidney on the same side. A dark purple color in this area indicates pyelonephritis.

12. Area of reproductive organs

In males, bulging skin in this area in a dark color and with rough lines indicates hypertrophy of the prostate gland. Red alternating with white or dark red indicates prostatitis.

In females, the presence of one (or several) round (or rod-like) spot or patch on certain parts of this area indicates a uterine myoma in the corresponding portion of the uterus. The presence of a white bulging patch with rough lines in the center of this area indicates intrauterine chronic inflammation (endometritis), but it may also appear in women with a intrauterine device in their uterus. If the skin of the white spots and patches is thickened, the endometrium is also thickened (hyperplastic). If a red color in this area is mixed with some white or coffee tint, then damp-heat has accumulated in the uterus and patients may discharge yellow or red leukorrhea. A red alternating with white color in bulging skin of this area on one hand indicates inflammation of the uterine appendages on the same side. The presence of an edematous or vascular prominence (no subcutaneous blood vessels) in this area on one side indicates an ovarian cyst on the same side.

13. Trachea area

This is the area that indicates the condition and diseases of the trachea and its main bronchi. A prominence in this area usually indicates bronchitis. Red in this area indicates congestion of the trachea in febrile diseases, and patients may suffer from dry cough and difficulty in coughing up sputum. The presence of a red prominence in this area indicates diseases caused by damp-heat, causing patients to spit up yellow sputum with sticky lumps. Red over a flat skin in this area indicates dry cough without sputum caused by dry heat. The presence of some red and white alternating nodules indicates suppurative bronchitis. White over a depressed skin in this area indicates deficiency of lung qi or Feiwei (a consumptive disease of lung, similar to pulmonary tuberculosis). The presence of some small dark coffee or purple pointed nodules with flocculent and infiltrating margins of the skin in a coffee color probably indicates cancers.

14. Area of left chest (lung)

The holographic spots corresponding to the left chest, lung, bronchus and breast are all distributed in this area. Small, dark, round and hard nodules in this area usually indicate the calcified foci of pulmonary tuberculosis. Red spread all over this area indicates pneumonia caused by lung heat. In the right half of this area next to the trachea area, an irregular papule in a brownish yellow or coffee color indicates chronic bronchitis. A papule similar to a blood vessel (not really a blood vessel) in this area indicates bronchiectasis. The presence of a horizontal brown bar similar to a small callus between both chest (lung) areas, along the base of the trachea area and just above the waist area indicates pulmonary emphysema.

15. Area of right chest (lung)

Observation diagnosis in this area is similar to that in the area of left chest (lung), except for the difference in sides of their corresponding organs.

16. Waist area

The presence of some small pits in the segment of the heaven line [heart line] within this area indicates trauma of the waist or deformity of lumbar vertebrae in the corresponding location. White (sometimes on bulging skin) along both sides of the heaven line indicates lumbago and soreness of waist. The whiter the skin in this area looks, the more severe the pain and soreness the patient may suffer from. The presence of a dominant red color alternating with some white tint indicates lumbago caused by trauma or muscular strain in the corresponding region of the waist. Blue blood vessels appearing in the center or in the heaven line of this white area indicate lumbago due to attack of coldness and poor blood supply.

17. Spleen area

The whole spleen area is evenly depressed. Flat skin in a white, grayish white or whitish blue color indicates deficiency or deficient-coldness of spleen. If the area is much more depressed, and the skin is bright white and the subcutaneous tissue is dark or light coffee in color, the spleen may be already excised or atrophic. Bulging skin with a yellow, yellowish brown (callus-like) or light coffee color indicates splenomegaly (enlargement of spleen) or deficiency of spleen (impairment of function) for a long period of time.

18. Gallbladder area

The presence of a red patch with clear white margins in the center of the gallbladder area indicates congestion or inflammation of the gallbladder and biliary ducts caused by heat in gallbladder. White bulging skin over this area indicates gallbladder colic. Red alternating with white in the bulging gallbladder area indicates inflammation of gallbladder or biliary ducts. White or bluish-white bulging skin with red borders in this area indicates acute cholecystitis. The presence of some hard nodules on white bulging skin indicates gallstone of the granular type; and the presence of irregular dark spots underneath white bulging skin indicates gallstone of the sandy type.

19. Area of (upper, middle and lower) abdomen

The stomach, liver and spleen are located in the upper abdomen, therefore, the diseases of these organs may show some visible signs in this area. For example, in the central region of this area, bulging skin in a dominant white color alternating with a reddish tint indicates distension of the stomach. The presence of some spots, patches or nodules of yellowish brown (callus-like) color in the corresponding regions of this area indicates tuberculosis of the intestine, tuberculosis of the peritoneum, intestinal polyps, chronic colitis or constipation. If the skin over the whole hypothenar prominence is red in color with some dark red spots and patchs, patients may have heat accumulated in their abdomen.

20. Area for dreaminess

The presence of pigmented black areas of pigmentation, a wart or scar in this area on the lateral side of the index finger certainly indicates dreaminess. A pure white color or a white color alternating with some reddish tint in this area also indicates dreaminess.

21 Area for insomnia

White color in this area indicates insomnia. Nodules in a pure white color or with a reddish tint in this area also indicate insomnia. A pure white or a white color alternating with some reddish tint over the whole proximal segment of the index finger indicates sleepiness due to deficiency of qi and blood and poor supply of cerebral blood.

22. Area for fatigue

White alternating with a reddish tint in this area indicates a general weakness due to insufficiency of sleep and rest. In patients with both dreaminess and insomnia, the fatigue is due to the low quality of their sleep; and in patients with sleepiness, the fatigue is a symptom of neurasthenia and weak physique.

23. Liver area

Bulging skin in the triangular liver area indicates enlargement of liver. The color white in this area indicates deficiency or stagnation of liver qi. Dark gray and bluish black color in the whole liver area and its neighboring areas indicates bad mood and mental depression. Dark blue skin or some white spots on the red skin of this area indicates hepatitis. At the same time, if some blue blood vessels can be seen underneath the skin, the clinical course of the hepatitis is of long standing. If a bright white color is evenly distributed all over the areas of liver, spleen, stomach, kidney and reproductive organs, patients suffer from liver cirrhosis.

24. Area for deficiency of qi

White alternating with a red color in this area indicates shortness of breath with repeated deep breath and sighing. If the face, ears, and lips (even the whole palm) are all white in color in addition to this area on the hand, patients may also suffer from anemia and malnutrition besides deficiency of Zhongjiao qi.

25. Heart area

In this area, the presence of a bulging prominence covered with a thin layer of shiny skin indicates cardiac hypertrophy or local enlargement of heart. If the whole thenar prominence is swollen, thickened, and purple or dark blue in color and some white and red spots or patchs are alternately and irregularly scattered underneath the skin, patients may suffer from palpitations of the heart, tachycardia or cardiac arrhythmia due to anoxia of heart muscles or viral myocarditis. A red color in the heart area (usually in the right heart area) and spread over the whole thenar prominence indicates excessiveness of heart fire.

26. Area for poor blood supply

The presence of some white spots on depressed skin of this area indicates poor blood supply to heart. The presence of some bluish-white bulging spots in this area indicates angina pectoris.

27. Area for edema

A pure white color or white color alternating with a reddish tint indicates edema due to restriction of general blood circulation. If the white color spreads to the area of left ventricle, patients may suffer from hypertrophy or enlargement of left ventricle.

28. Bladder area

Pure white color or a white color alternating with a reddish tint on the bulging skin of this area indicates a downward pouring of damp-heat that will cause a discharge of yellow urine with a bad odor. A red or pink color over the whole bladder area indicates blood congestion in the bladder or congestive inflammation of the bladder.

29. Skin area

White or a white prominence in this area indicates pruritus (itching of skin) or urticaria of the skin in a corresponding location. A callus-like bulging patch with a light coffee or dark color in this area indicates eczema, dermatitis or psoriasis. A dark yellow prominence indicates allergic skin diseases or allergic dermatitis. White, shiny and smooth skin over this area indicates anemia and pruritus caused by senility or by diabetes mellitus.

30. Area for rheumatism

A bluish white or bluish purple color in this area indicates the common cold caused by wind-cold pathogen. Dark purple or purplish gray color with a bluish tint in this area indicates rheumatism.

31. Anus area

The presence of a small papule or nodule around the tip of the finger indicates internal and external hemorrhoids in a corresponding location in the area of the anus. The presence of some subcutaneous stripes in a dark red, purplish red or coffee color indicates anal fissures.

32. Rectum area

Red alternating with a white tint or a white color alternating with a red tint in this area indicates proctitis. In this area, the presence of a blister with some fluid of coffee or dark red color and a red halo around it indicates cancer of the rectum with metastasis through the lymphatic system. The presence of several nodules of dark yellow or coffee color in this area indicates polyps or tumors in the rectum that can cause chronic diarrhea for many years.

33. Area of the left shoulder and arm

White spots and patches in this area indicate diseases of the left shoulder with pain. The presence of some blue blood vessels passing through this area indicates blood stasis in the blood vessels around the left shoulder to indicate that patients may suffer numbness, weakness and aching in the left arm.

34. Area of the right shoulder and arm

Observation diagnosis in this area for diseases of the right shoulder and arm is similar to that mentioned in the "Area of the left shoulder and arm."

35. Area of the left ear

If the skin over this area is depressed, patients may suffer from otopiesis (inward depression of the eardrum membrane), hearing impairment, hypersensitivity to sound of high or low frequency (usually to high frequency) and tinnitus of the left ear. White or bluish white spots and patches in this area indicate acute otitis media with pain in the left ear. The presence of some fine blue blood vessels beneath the skin of this area (often accompanied with inward depression of the left drum membrane) indicates impairment of hearing and tinnitus (nervous deafness and tinnitus) and hypersensitivity to high-frequency sounds.

36. Area of the right ear

Observation diagnosis for diseases of the right ear is similar to that in the "Area of the left ear."

37. Spine and back areas

According to the location of a prominence or hypertrophic nodule on the extensor tendon of the middle finger, a diagnosis of hypertrophy and hyperosteogeny of its corresponding spinal vertebra can be made. The metacarpophalangeal joint of middle finger is defined as the referred location of the Dazhui (DU 14) point on the neck and a brown or brownish black color appearing at or beside the joint indicates a suffering of pain in or beside the cervical spine. The presence of an engorged blood vessel around or beside the joint indicates arteriosclerosis of vertebrobasilar or cerebral artery. The presence of some blue (usually) or purplish red (occasionally) subcutaneous blood vessels around the joint indicates blood stasis and deficiency of blood supply in the vertebrobasilar and cerebral arteries.

38. Area of occiput of head

A watery white color hidden beneath the skin in this area indicates hydrocephalus in the occiput of head, and patients may be suffering from Meniere's syndrome with dizziness, nausea and vomiting. The small blue and bluish gray blood vessels underneath the skin indicate insufficient blood supply and cerebral anoxia to cause dizziness. A white tint around the subcutaneous blood vessels indicates headache as a result of poor blood supply or some external trauma.

III. Remarks

1. The hands should not be washed or rubbed before making an observation diagnosis because those actions might interfere with the reliability of the diagnosis. Hands should be diagnosed under a natural light, rather than lamplight. Direct sunlight also is not an adequate light source.

2. Both physicians and patients must keep their minds calm, their thoughts in order and their attention concentrated when they

are making a hand observation diagnosis.

3. To guarantee the reliability of a hand diagnosis, physicians must have mastered the correct locations of holographic areas of all organs and parts of the body.

4. Hand diagnosis must be guided by the five-element theory, yin and yang theory and modern theories of Western medicine. Positive findings must be carefully analyzed and evaluated to distinguish between major and minor ones. The balance between yin and yang as well as the connections between superficial phenomena and internal pathogenesis must be emphasized to make a correct diagnosis.

CHAPTER 5
HAND ACUPUNCTURE THERAPY INTRODUCTION

Section 1 Therapeutic Methods Applied to Acupuncture Points on the Hand

Therapeutic methods that simulate acupuncture points or areas on the hand can adjust the functions of the whole body and prevent or treat diseases. Many therapies exist, but only several common methods will be discussed as follows.

I. Acupuncture

In this treatment, acupuncture needles simulate points on the hand to treat diseases.

1. Selection of needles

Four types (No. 26, 28, 30, and 32) of regular acupuncture needles with a length of 0.5-1.0 cun are usually used in clinical practice.

2. Therapeutic method

(1) Insertion technique: Because the points on the hand are sensitive to pain, a pricking technique is used to insert the needle. With the handle of the needle held firmly between the thumb and index finger, the needle quickly and precisely pierces the point through a

sudden thrusting movement applied by the wrist. The action must be steady, accurate and quick to produce only very brief and mild pain.

(2) Depth of insertion: Needles are usually inserted to a depth of 1-2 cm, depending where the point lies on the anatomy. The needle may be inserted to a deeper level in patients with excessive or heat syndrome and emergent or painful diseases. The insertion of the needle must be very shallow in weak patients, children and the elderly.

(3) Direction of insertion: The needle may be inserted vertically, on a slant or horizontally.

(4) Retention and removal of needle: In general, the needle can remain in the point for 20-30 minutes. For patients with persistent or painful diseases, the time the needle remains inserted may be prolonged from 30 to 60 minutes, but in children the needle should be removed immediately without any retention. Throughout the retention period, needles are manipulated to reinforce the stimulation at ten-minute intervals. For removal, needles may be pulled out quickly or with a twisting motion, but in any case the tip of needle should be quickly exit the skin. The spot of the prick should be pressed with a piece of sterilized cotton ball to prevent bleeding.

3. Points for attention

(1) Before acupuncture is used, both the skin of the patient and the needles should be carefully sterilized to prevent infection.

(2) Acupuncture is contraindicated in patients who are either in extreme hunger or have eaten too much; who are overtired, drunk, or physically weak; who have a nervous disposition or have just recovered from serious illness. In these cases, acupuncture may cause fainting.

(3) It is also contraindicated in pregnant women.

(4) Acupuncture should not be applied to points on the skin with frostbite or inflammation because it may spread infection.

(5) Before treatment, patients should be asked about any history of repeated attacks of dizziness, chest distress or nausea, and the practitioners should be alert for the appearance of a pale complexion

and profuse sweating as signs during treatment. If signs of fainting are detected, the needles should be removed immediately and patient should be in a lying position with the head in a lower position in a room with good ventilation. Patients with mild fainting need not receive any particular management; they should recover after a few minutes of rest. In severe cases, the oxygen or a hypodermic injection of a respiratory stimulant may be needed to revive the patient.

II. Bleeding Therapy

This therapy causes bleeding by pricking the acupuncture points on the hand with a three-edged needle or regular acupuncture needles.

1. Needle

As the Fengzhen (sharp needle) of the ancient "9 needles," the three-edged needle is made of stainless steel in a length of 6 cm. The needle body is thick and round in shape and its tip is in the shape of a pointed prism with three sharp edges.

2. Therapeutic method

(1) The distal segment of the finger for application of the treatment should be thoroughly rubbed to cause congestion, and the skin should be sterilized.

(2) The three-edged needle is held by the physician to quickly prick the acupuncture point for 1-3 mm in depth, and then 3-5 drops of blood are squeezed out of the small hole. Finally, a dry cotton ball is applied and pressed over the hole to stop the bleeding. The treatment is applied once every other day, but it may be applied once or twice a day in emergency patients.

3. Indications

The treatment can produce a therapeutic effect to open orifices, lower fever, promote blood circulation, lessen swelling, relieve pain and promote circulation of qi in the meridians and collaterals. This treats high and low fever, inflammation, hypertension, vertigo, dizziness, eye diseases, acute and chronic hepatitis, skin diseases and sore throat.

4. Points for attention

(1) The procedure of rubbing the skin around the acupuncture points before treatment is very important to cause local blood congestion to produce enough bleeding for a good therapeutic result.

(2) The skin of hand must be thoroughly sterilized, and the treatment must be carried out following the general rules of sterilization.

(3) The prick of the three-edged needle should not be very deep.

(4) The amount of bleeding should be adequate, depending upon the severity of diseases and physique (weak or strong) of patients. Generally speaking, the amount of bleeding should not be very much.

(5) This treatment is contraindicated in women during menstrual period and patients with diseases prone for bleeding, such as hemophilia, aplastic anemia and primary thrombocytopenia.

III. Moxibustion

This therapeutic method prevents and treats diseases by applying heat to stimulate the points on the hand with the burnt moxa and other herbs.

1. Materials for moxibustion

In general, moxa cones and moxa rolls are used for moxibustion. The moxa cones are handmade of moxa in the shape of a cone. Moxa rolls are prepared with moxa and paper of mulberry bark in long cylindrical paper rolls secured by glued edges.

2. Therapeutic method

(1) Moxa cone method: A moxa cone is put on a selected acupuncture point and its tip is lit. After two-thirds of the cone has been burned, the residual moxa is replaced by a new cone to repeat the treatment. In general, several or more than 10 cones are used for a treatment to turn the local skin hot and flushed.

(2) Moxa roll method: After lighting one end of a moxa roll, the ignited end is held above a selected point at a distance far enough away from the skin to avoid burning but close enough to produce a

comfortable and warm sensation.

3. Indications

Moxibustion can warm meridians, dispel cold pathogens, relax muscles, remove stagnation in collaterals, relieve pain and reduce swelling to treat cold syndrome, deficiency syndrome, pain syndrome and particularly the Bi-syndrome.

4. Points for attention

(1) Care should be taken to avoid burning the skin during the application of moxibustion. If the skin is burned and blisters form, the damaged skin should be treated according to regular burn treatments.

(2) Moxibustion should be used with care in extremely nervous people, patients with severe heart and kidney disease, and pregnant women.

IV. Aqua-acupuncture

This method — also called acupuncture-point injection therapy — treats diseases by injecting Western drugs or Chinese herbs into acupuncture points.

1. Drugs and herbs for injection

(1) Western drugs: Vitamin B_1, B_{12} and C, 0.5% novocaine, placental globulin, brain tissue fluid, saline solution, distilled water, dexamethasone and desoxycortisone.

(2) Chinese herbs: Injection solutions of Danggui (Chinese Angelica root), Huanglian (Coptidis rhizome), Huangqi (Astragali root), Banlangen (Isatidis root) and Danshen (Salvia root).

2. Therapeutic method

(1) Drugs or herbs are prescribed as appropriate for the diagnosed condition.

(2) The skin around the points is sterilized for injection of the solution.

(3) A syringe of 1-2 ml with No. 4 needle is used to inject the solution.

(4) A solution of 0.5 ml is injected subcutaneously into each point.

(5) After injection of the solution, a cotton ball is used to press the puncture point to control bleeding and leaking of the solution.

(6) Course of treatment: One to three acupuncture points are selected for injections; the treatment is applied once every other day, and one therapeutic course consists of 10 treatments. A one-week rest should be arranged between successive courses.

3. Points for attention

(1) The skin around the points as well as the instruments used for injection must be carefully sterilized to prevent infection.

(2) For injection of drugs or herbs capable of inducing allergic reaction, a skin test should be done before the treatment.

(3) Before injection of drugs, their directions on pharmacological actions, contraindications, production date and duration of efficacy must be read and thoroughly understood.

(4) Aqua-acupuncture is contraindicated in pregnant women, and it should be prescribed with care to weak and elderly patients.

(5) Alternative points should be selected in groups for each treatment in succession.

V. Electroacupuncture

After insertion of a needle into an acupuncture point, a weak electrical current is sent through the needle to prevent and treat diseases. The intensity of electrical stimulation may be adjusted for achieving a better therapeutic effect according to the nature and severity of the disease. This is an effective therapy to treat asthma and pain.

1. Therapeutic methods

(1) Needles are inserted into selected points in succession.

(2) Before the electricity of the electroacupuncture machine is turned on, the output current of the machine is turned down to "0." The conducting wire is connected to the needle handles and the

output current is gradually turned up to an adequate level tolerable to the patient.

(3) Before ending the treatment, the electrical current is turned down to "0" again, and then the machine is turned off. After the wire is disconnected, the needles are removed.

(4) In each treatment, electrical stimulation is applied to one to two groups of points, each group having six points, and maintained for 10-15 minutes. The treatment is applied once a day or once every other day. A therapeutic course consists of 10 such treatments.

(5) In general, the duration of the electrical stimulation may be longer in younger patients and patients with pain or persistent diseases, but it should be shorter in children and weaker patients.

2. Points for attention

(1) Electrical current must be gradually increased; a sudden surge could produce intolerable discomfort.

(2) The positive and negative poles of the conducting wire should be connected to two points on the same hand, rather than on both hands.

(3) Electroacupuncture is contraindicated in the case of pregnant women and weak patients.

VI. Photo-acupuncture

Photo-acupuncture — also called laser irradiation therapy — applies laser stimulation to hand acupuncture points. A gas laser therapy apparatus of low potential, such as a HeNe [Helium Neon] laser apparatus or Ar laser apparatus, is used in the treatment. The channels of the new brands of laser machines have been increased from 2-4 to 10-15. Therefore, the scope of application of this technology has been greatly widened. Today, the HeNe laser transmitter is widely used in clinical practice.

1. Therapeutic methods

(1) Before applying laser irradiation, the apparatus should be carefully checked and the pointers of all scales turned to the "0"

position. After the electricity is turned on and adjusted to an adequate level, a steady red laser beam can be generated to apply to the selected points.

(2) Laser irradiation is applied for 20-30 minutes, once a day or once every other day with 10 times of irradiation making a therapeutic course.

(3) After the treatment is finished, the electrical potential is turned down to the "0" level and the electrical source of the apparatus is turned off.

2. Points for attention

(1) The laser transmitter should be kept in good repair to prevent dust, moisture and shock.

(2) If the apparatus is not used for a long time, it should be regularly turned on and warmed up for one hour each month.

(3) Laser irradiation is contraindicated in patients very sensitive to the laser ray.

(4) A laser beam absolutely must not be used to irradiate the pupil of eye.

VII. Massage

Massage may be applied at various points, areas and parts of the hand to prevent and treat various diseases. It is a simple and useful therapeutic method that anyone can use to improve health and treat both acute and chronic diseases.

1. Therapeutic methods

(1) Pressing with the thumb: The thumb is used to press the points and small holographic areas of the hand to produce a tolerable sensation of soreness and distension. The pressing and rotating maneuvers may be combined in this application.

(2) Pushing maneuver with thumb: The thumb is used to push the big holographic areas, fingers or the whole palm and dorsum of hand.

(3) In each treatment, the massage is performed for 20-30

minutes, once a day or once every other day. A therapeutic course consists of 5-10 treatments.

2. Points for Attention

(1) For patients of chronic diseases, the massage must be applied continuously day-by-day until a good therapeutic result is achieved.

(2) Performance of massage is forbidden on patients with inflammation or frostbite on their hands.

(3) The location on the hand must be accurate for the massage to produce a good therapeutic effect.

VIII. Magnetic Therapy

This method — also called magnet adhesion therapy — uses a magnetic field to stimulate the acupuncture points on hand for prevention and treatment of diseases. Magnetic energy may be transmitted into the human body to promote metabolism, improve blood circulation, adjust nervous functions, reduce inflammation and prevent infection. Therefore, it may be used to reduce inflammation and swelling, relieve pain and itching, control diarrhea and asthma, and produce sedative and hypotensive effects.

1. Therapeutic methods

According to the disease, small magnets can be stuck directly on the acupuncture points on one or both hands with an adhesive. No more than four magnets should be used, and they should be replaced with new ones after three to five days of use.

2. Points for attention

(1) The number of magnets used in a treatment should be limited, otherwise interference between different magnetic fields may lessen the therapeutic effect.

(2) Magnetic therapy should be stopped in a timely fashion if palpitations, nausea, dizziness or weakness should come on the patient during treatment.

(3) An anti-allergic adhesive plaster should be used to apply the magnets.

Section 2 Hand Acupuncture Therapy Indications and Contraindications

Hand acupuncture therapy can be used to treat various diseases of internal medicine; surgery; gynecology; pediatrics; ear, nose and throat; and dermatology.

I. Indications of Hand Acupuncture Therapy

1. Diseases with pain
(1) Inflammatory pain: Pharyngitis, cholecystitis, mastitis, rheumatic arthritis, and prostatitis.
(2) Traumatic pain: Sprain and strains, bone fracture, joint dislocation, and stiff neck.
(3) Neurotic pain: Neurotic headache, trigeminal neuralgia, neuralgia sciatica, and herpes zoster.
(4) Pain of tumors: Pain caused by tumors in the late stage.
2. Diseases with inflammation: Acute and chronic conjunctivitis, electric ophthalmitis, periodontitis, otitis media, tonsillitis, bronchitis, pneumonia, pleuritis, gastritis, enteritis, cystitis, and adnexitis.
3. Allergic diseases: Allergic rhinitis, asthma, allergic colitis, drug rash, and rheumatoid arthritis.
4. Diseases with endocrine dysfunction: Simple goiter, hyperthyroidism, diabetes mellitus, obesity, and menopausal syndrome.
5. Diseases due to bodily dysfunction: Dizziness, cardiac arrhythmia, hypertension, disorder of the stomach and intestine, polyhidrosis, irregular menses, urine incontinence, neurasthenia, sexual disorders, and functional uterine bleeding.
6. Other diseases: Lumbago and pain in leg, cervical syndrome, frozen shoulder, numbness of the limbs, hyperosteogeny, indigestion, and sequelae of brain injury.

II. Contraindications of Hand Acupuncture Therapy

1. Application of strong stimulation is prohibited for patients with severe heart diseases.

2. Hand acupuncture is contraindicated in patients with serious organic lesions, severe anemia, and hemophilia.

3. The therapy cannot be applied to patients with temporary frostbite, ulcers, inflammation and eczema on the hand.

4. Acupuncture is an inadequate treatment for women who are in the 40th-90th days of pregnancy — particularly when it is applied to the holographic area of the abdomen or lumbar and sacral spine. The therapy is contraindicated to treat the pregnant women of habitual abortion.

5. The acupuncture should be applied with care to women during their menstrual period.

Section 3 Principles for Selection of Acupuncture Points and Holographic Areas

The principles for selecting the points for hand acupuncture therapy are similar to those involved in regular acupuncture, so the principles of differential diagnosis and treatment of syndromes are particularly important to guide the practice of this therapy for achieving a good therapeutic result. First of all, the principles of the four diagnostic methods should be followed to make a correct diagnosis of diseases, and then the adequate points and areas should be selected on the basis of their functions and indications to compose a reasonable prescription. The important principles for selection of points and areas are mentioned as follows.

I. According to the Involved Organs

For application of local acupuncture therapy of the holographic embryo system on the hand, the holographic area on the hand corresponding to the involved organ should be selected. For example, the gallbladder area is selected for the treatment of acute or chronic cholecystitis and the area for insomnia is chosen for the treatment of insomnia.

II. According to the Theories of Zangfu and Jingluo in Traditional Chinese Medicine

As mentioned in the Traditional Chinese Medicine classics: "Where the meridian passes through, there lies a lesion curable by acupuncture applied on the points of that meridian; and, if any organ is related to that meridian, the lesion of that organ is curable by acupuncture on the points of this meridian."

Therefore, acupuncture points on the hand three yin and three yang meridians are selected to treat diseases of their related organs. For example, the Shaoshang (LU 11) point is selected to treat nasal bleeding and sore throat; and the Laogong (PC 8) is used to treat the febrile diseases, vomiting and hiccups.

III. According to Specific Functions of Acupuncture Points

The principle is followed to select some specific and extra meridianal points on the hand for clinical practice. For example, the point for shoulder pain is selected to treat shoulder pain and the point for diarrhea is used to treat diarrhea.

IV. According to Basic Theories of Traditional Chinese Medicine

The principle "to analyze the syndrome (clinical manifestations of disease) for discovery of its pathogenic factors and to discover the pathogenic factors for treatment of disease" should be followed to select acupuncture points. For example, because "the eye is an external opening of the liver" and the inflammation of eye with redness and swelling is due to upward flaming of liver fire, the liver area and point for high fever are selected to treat conjunctivitis of the eyelid. In addition, the basic principles of "the simultaneous treatment of both superficial and internal disturbances in the patient," "the mutual transformation of the ascending and descending (pathogenic factors or therapeutic effect)," and "the complementation between fire and water" should also be considered and followed in clinical practice.

The principles for selection of points and areas mentioned above are different from each other, but they are also closely related to each other. Therefore, they should easily be adopted in combination so that fewer but more efficient points and areas of the hand can be selected to achieve the best therapeutic results.

Section 4 Treatment of Fainting Caused by Needling in Hand Acupuncture Therapy

I. Causes of Fainting During Needling

Fainting can often happen in patients the first time they receive needling during acupuncture treatment, particularly when they are very nervous, sensitive to pain or prone to fainting; and it may also happen in patients with hunger and hypoglycemia. The strong stimulation produced by an unskillful manipulation by the clinician, high voltage of electrical current in electroacupuncture, wrong locality of an acupuncture point, inadequate posture assumed by the patient over a prolonged time while receiving treatment, and a combined therapy with multiple management are also common causes of fainting during needling.

II. Manifestations of Fainting During Needling

During the initial application of acupuncture or as the needles are retained, patients may suddenly develop symptoms of cerebral ischemia such as dizziness, blurred vision, chest distress and sweating in mild cases. In moderate cases, symptoms that may occur include heart palpitations, nausea, vomiting, pale complexion, very weak pulse and cold limbs. And in serious cases, patients may develop an ice-cold body and limbs, experience profuse sweating or a quick drop of blood pressure, or even slip into a coma. In clinical practice, the incidence of fainting during needling is about one percent, but the occurrence of the severe type is very rare.

III. Treatment of Fainting

Patients with mild fainting should be given some hot water to drink and put into a lying position. The clinician should talk to the patient to explain and console to relieve any nervousness, and then the fainting attack caused by needling may gradually go away. In moderate and severe attacks, patients should be put immediately into the Trendelenburg's position with their heads at a low level after the needles and pillow are all removed. Strong pressure can be applied at the Renzhong (DU 26) point with the clinician's finger, and a needling stimulation can be applied at the subcortical or adrenal point of ear. If that does not work, oxygen or an injection of adrenaline or coramine can be administered.

IV. Prevention of Fainting During Needling

Before starting acupuncture treatment, a clear and detailed explanation about its safe and non-traumatic nature should be made to assuage any nervousness. Treatment should never be forced on patients who do not understand the procedure or purpose of the treatment. Old and weak patients as well as those with a past history of fainting should be put into a prone position to receive treatment, fewer points and areas should be selected for acupuncture, and the needling stimulation should be milder in intensity. Treatment should never be done on patients with an empty stomach, with hypoglycemia, who are overtired or who have been sweating profusely. To guarantee a smooth acupuncture treatment, patients always should be put into a comfortable position so that they can tolerate needle retention over a long time.

CHAPTER 6

CLINICAL APPLICATION OF HAND ACUPUNCTURE THERAPY

Section 1 Common Diseases of Internal Medicine

I. Diseases of the Respiratory System

1. Bronchitis
[Pathogenesis and clinical manifestations]

Bronchitis of the acute and chronic type is an inflammatory disease of the trachea and bronchi caused by a viral or bacterial infection, physical or chemical irritation or allergic reaction. In an acute attack, the onset of the disease is sudden with patients suffering from symptoms of upper respiratory tract infection such as chills, low fever, headache, throat pain, cough, and even shortness of breath with wheezing in the case of bronchial spasm. The patients with chronic bronchitis may suffer from a persistent cough and spit sputum, sometimes mixed with blood.

[Hand diagnosis]

In patients with acute bronchitis, some white or red nodules may be scattered over the trachea area on the hand, and the white and red nodules are distributed alternately in patients with severe cough and expectoration. In patients with chronic bronchitis, the yellow or dark brown nodules may be scattered over rough skin in the trachea area. In the acute stage, white spots may also appear in the nose and pharynx areas.

[Selection of points]

First-choice points: Point for asthma and cough and Yuji (LU 10).

Secondary points: Shaoshang (LU 11), point for pain of throat and teeth, and trachea area.

[Therapeutic method]

Regular acupuncture is applied at the point for asthma and cough, Yuji point and point for throat; bleeding therapy is applied at the Shaoshang point; and the pressing maneuver of massage is applied with the thumb at the trachea area.

[Remarks]

In patients with acute bronchitis and severe infection, antibiotics and Chinese herbs should be prescribed.

2. Bronchial asthma

[Pathogenesis and clinical manifestations]

This allergic disease is characterized by paroxysmal attacks of bronchiole spasm, mucosal edema and lung congestion. About half of patients have a family history of the disease. Attacks are usually induced through inhaling allergic antigens (pollens and dust); eating fish, shrimp or egg, or having an infection of the respiratory tract. Some preliminary symptoms may appear before the onset of the disease. These include cough, chest distress, itching in the nose and sneezing. Later, patients may suffer from more severe symptoms such as severe chest distress, dyspnea, tightness in the chest, forced to stay in a sitting position and even cyanosis and cold sweat in critical patients. Each attack may last for hours or a few days.

[Hand diagnosis]

A dark blue color may appear over an uneven skin in the center of the trachea area. Some findings similar to those of bronchitis can be found in patients with a severe infection in the lung.

[Selection of points]

First-choice points: New point for asthma and Yuji (LU 10).

Secondary points: Shaoshang (LU 11) and trachea area.

[Therapeutic methods]

Regular acupuncture is applied at the new point for asthma and Yuji point. The needle is inserted at a slant into the Yuji point toward the center of the palm for 1-1.5 cun. Bleeding therapy is applied at Shaoshang point, and the pressing maneuver of massage with the thumb is applied in the trachea area.

[Remarks]

In patients with a severe attack of asthma, oxygen and spasmolytic drugs should be administered.

3. Pneumonia

[Pathogenesis and clinical manifestations]

Pneumonia is an acute alveolar infection of the lung, caused by pneumococci and most prevalent in the winter and spring. The dominant symptoms of the disease are chills, high fever, chest pain, cough and spitting of rusty sputum. It is common in youths.

[Hand diagnosis]

In the area of chest and lung, some spots are found in red or a red alternating with white, with clear borders.

[Selection of points]

First-choice points: Hegu (LI 4), point of lung, point for chest pain, and point for asthma and cough.

Secondary points: Shixuan (EX-UE 11), area of the chest and lung and trachea area.

[Therapeutic methods]

Regular acupuncture is applied at all first-choice points; bleeding therapy is applied at the Shixuan point; and massage or application of magnets is performed in the trachea area and area of chest and lung as a supplemental treatment.

[Remarks]

Seriously ill patients should be treated with the antibiotics and Chinese herbs as well as the hand acupuncture therapy mentioned above.

4. Bronchiectasis

[Pathogenesis and clinical manifestation]

Bronchiectasis is a disease of the bronchi with abscesses or irreversible anatomical dilatation and deformation of the lung. The disease is usually a complication involving acute infectious lung diseases that either have not been treated with a satisfactory therapy or that have been caused by pulmonary tuberculosis, lung abscesses, chronic bronchitis or bronchial asthma. Common symptoms include repeated attacks of coughing, spitting of sputum and spitting of blood caused by the dilatation and rupture of bronchial walls. X-rays of the chest may show increased lung markings and orbital and curly shadows.

[Hand diagnosis]

In patients with bronchiectasis, some dark red nodules may appear in the trachea area and the holographic area of the bronchus. Fresh red spots in this area indicate fresh hemoptysis and the brown spots indicate a history of hemoptysis in the past.

[Selection of points]

First-choice points: Yuji (LU 10), Laogong (PC 8) and point of lung.

Secondary points: Trachea area, lung area and point for cough.

[Therapeutic methods]

Regular acupuncture is applied at the point of lung, Yuji and Laogong points with the needle slanting from Yuji to Laogong point for application of a purging maneuver. Bleeding therapy with a three-edged needle is performed at the point of lung after regular acupuncture has been applied. The massage or magnet therapy is performed in the trachea and lung areas and at the point for cough as a supplemental treatment.

[Remarks]

Bronchiectasis is a stubborn disease resistant to treatment. Therefore, a combined therapy of the Western medicine and Traditional Chinese Medicine should be adopted to treat patients with severe hemoptysis and infection. At the same time, patients should be put in a Trendelenburg's position for expectorating sputum and fluid accumulated in the bronchial cavities.

5. Pulmonary emphysema

[Pathogenesis and clinical manifestations]

As a complication of many chronic diseases of the lung, pulmonary emphysema is a disease involving reduced elasticity of lung tissues, increase of lung volume and impairment of respiratory function due to an over-inflation and expansion of the bronchioli, alveolar ducts and alveoli of the lung. Chronic obstructive pulmonary emphysema is a common type of the disease. Besides the coughing with sputum associated with the primary disease, another symptom is a gradually increased air hunger. In the early stages, patients may have shortness of breath during or after some exertion, but later on they may suffer from dyspnea and cyanosis even during rest. The disease can be exacerbated in winter or after a severe lung infection.

[Hand diagnosis]

Some yellow nodules may appear in the trachea area and the skin over the lung area is covered with some prominent and rough dark blue striae.

[Selection of points]

First-choice points: Yuji (LU 10), point for asthma and point of lung.

Secondary points: Bronchus area and area of chest and lung (bilateral).

[Therapeutic methods]

Regular acupuncture is applied at Yuji point and point for asthma; the three-edged needle is used to bleed 3-4 drops of blood from the point of lung. At the same time, the pressing massage with thumb is performed in the bronchus area and bilateral areas of chest and lung.

[Remarks]

Patients must try their best to maintain their health, prevent any attack of the common cold and control lung infection. A significant supply of oxygen should be given to patients with severe cyanosis.

II. Disease of the Cardiovascular System

1. Hypertensive disease

[Pathogenesis and clinical manifestation]

This is a common syndrome with dizziness, headache and uneasiness caused by systemic high-blood pressure. Hand acupuncture therapy can relieve the symptoms of both primary and secondary hypertension in the early and middle stage, but a combined therapy with drugs should be administered to patients in the late stage.

[Hand diagnosis]

Some white, red, dark red or yellow nodules can be seen in the area for hypertension. Scattered white spots indicate hypertension of the first stage with a fluctuated blood pressure. A dense area of white spots indicates hypertension at the late stage with persistent high blood pressure, and the spots also may be found in the area for dizziness. Red or dark red spots indicate renal hypertension with very high blood pressure due to hyperactivity of liver yang over a long period of time. Yellow nodules indicate persistent hypertension.

[Selection of points]

First-choice points: Zhongchong (PC 9), Houxi (SI 3) and point of liver.

Secondary points: Shixuan (EX-UE 11), point for pain of vortex of head, area for hypertension and area for dizziness.

[Therapeutic methods]

Regular acupuncture is applied at the point of liver and Houxi point and bleeding therapy with a three-edged needle is applied at Zhongchong point. If this treatment does not work, bleeding therapy may again be applied at the Shixuan points. Massage or application of magnets is performed in the areas for hypertension and dizziness.

2. Hypotensive disease

[Pathogenesis and clinical manifestation]

In patients with hypotension, blood pressure may be lower than the normal range of 90 mmHg of systolic pressure and 40-50 mmHg of diastolic pressure. Major symptoms of the disease are dizziness, weakness and insomnia.

[Hand diagnosis]

A bright white color appears in the area for hypotension.

[Selection of points]

First-choice points: Point to raise blood pressure and area for hypotension.

Secondary points: Area for dizziness and area for insomnia.

[Therapeutic methods]

Regular acupuncture is applied at the point to raise blood pressure, and massage is performed in the areas for hypotension, dizziness and insomnia.

3. Coronary heart disease

[Pathogenesis and clinical manifestation]

This is a disease with ischemia and oxygen deficiency in the cardiac muscles caused by arteriosclerosis and induced by over fatigue, emotional disturbance, an overfull stomach or an attack of coldness. A major symptom of the disease is a sudden onset of a compressive and asphyxiating dull pain behind the upper, middle and lower segments of the sternum with a radiating pain spreading to the left shoulder, arm, little finger and ring finger. The pain may disappear after a few minutes rest or taking buccal nitroglycerine.

[Hand diagnosis]

In patients with coronary heart disease, a small hard varicose blood vessel can be seen in the center of the metacarpophalangeal crease of thumb. An irregular patch of red alternating with white is present in the heart area. Some white spots or pits may appear in the area for poor blood supply. Bluish white spots in this area indicate angina pectoris.

[Selection of points]

First-choice points: Shaofu (HT 8), Shaochong (HT 9) and point of heart.

Supplement points: Heart area and area for poor blood supply.

[Therapeutic methods]

Regular acupuncture is applied at Shaofu point; bleeding therapy is applied at Shaochong point; and massage is performed in the heart area and area for poor blood supply.

[Remarks]

The onset of the disease is sudden, so buccal nitroglycerine should be administered in time. Patients with severe cardiac infarction should be transported immediately to a hospital for resuscitation.

4. Heart neurosis

[Pathogenesis and clinical manifestations]

Heart neurosis is a disease of the heart caused by a disturbance in the nervous system, rather than an organic lesion in the heart. The disease is more common in women 20-40 years old. Common symptoms include dyspnea, palpitations of the heart, fatigue, precordial pain, vertigo, profuse sweating and insomnia — often exacerbated by over fatigue and mental stress.

[Hand diagnosis]

A string of blue spots are present in the heart area and on the radial side of the middle one-third of the extended segment of the midline of the thumb from its metacarpophalangeal crease to the palmar wrist crease. A white color appears over the area for insomnia.

[Selection of points]

First-choice points: Shaofu (HT 8), Guanchong (SJ 1), Laogong (PC 8) and heart area.

Secondary points: Area for insomnia and area for dizziness.

[Therapeutic methods]

Regular acupuncture is applied at Shaofu and Guanchong points, and massage or application of magnet therapy is performed in the areas for insomnia and dizziness and also at the Laogong point for calming the mind.

5. Cardiac arrhythmia

[Pathogenesis and clinical manifestations]

Common cardiac arrhythmia involving sinus arrhythmia, rapid

heart beat (tachycardia), abnormally slow heart beat (bradycardia), premature heart beat, atrial fibrillation, and atrioventricular block can be caused by dysfunction of the vegetative nervous system, coronary heart disease, myocarditis and rheumatic heart disease. Patients may suffer from heart palpitations, chest distress, shortness of breath and vertigo.

[Hand diagnosis]

The lateral portion of the heart area may show a red, dark red or blue color. A dark blue bulging blood vessel may also occur in this region. A red color indicates rapid heart beat, blue indicates abnormally slow heart beat, and a blue bulging blood vessel indicates a blockage.

[Selection of points]

Shaofu (HT 8) and Shaochong (HT 9), heart area and point of heart.

[Therapeutic methods]

Regular acupuncture is applied at Shaofu, Shaochong and point of heart; bleeding therapy is applied at Shaochong point; and massage or magnet therapy is performed in the heart area.

6. Myocarditis

[Pathogenesis and clinical manifestations]

This is an acute, subacute or chronic inflammation in local or diffused cardiac muscles as a complication of a general disease, including epidemic influenza, measles, chicken pox, and mumps. Patients with a mild type of the disease may suffer from palpitations of heart, chest distress, dull precordial pain and weakness; and patients with severe myocarditis may suffer from arrhythmia, heart failure and cardiac shock.

[Hand diagnosis]

The skin over the thenar prominence is swollen, thickened and purple or dark blue in color with one or some subcutaneous spots and patches of red alternating with white.

[Selection of points]

First-choice points: Shaochong (HT 9), Laogong (PC 8) and

heart area.

Secondary points: Point of heart, area for poor blood supply and Zhongchong (SJ 1).

[Therapeutic methods]

Bleeding therapy or a quick prick of an acupuncture needle (not retained in place) is applied at Shaochong, Zhongchong and point of heart, and massage with thumb is performed in the heart area and area for poor blood supply and at Laogong point.

[Remarks]

Patients with mild myocarditis can be cured by hand acupuncture therapy alone, but severe myocarditis must be treated in time through a combined therapy of Western medicine and Traditional Chinese Medicine. Patients with severe symptoms of heart failure and heart arrhythmia can only be saved through emergency treatment.

7. Chronic rheumatic heart disease

[Pathogenesis and clinical manifestations]

Chronic rheumatic heart disease with deformity of the cardiac valves is the result of acute rheumatic heart disease. The mitral and aortic valves of the heart are often involved to cause stenosis of the valve opening, valvular insufficiency or both in combination. Valvular lesions may produce hemodynamics, heart murmurs, cardiac insufficiency and congestive heart failure. Patients may suffer from palpitations of the heart, dyspnea, coughing and shortness of breath. The causes of rheumatic heart disease are still unknown, although it is thought closely related to rheumatic fever.

[Hand diagnosis]

Some dark red or dark blue spots are found in the area of mitral valve (near the metacarpophalangeal crease in the heart area), and a dark blue color appears in the area for rheumatism.

[Selection of points]

First-choice points: Shaochong (HT 9), Laogong (PC 8), point of heart and area for rheumatism.

Secondary points: Heart area and area of mitral valve.

[Therapeutic methods]

Regular acupuncture is applied at Shaochong, Laogong and point of heart, and massage with thumb or magnet therapy is performed in the heart area, area of mitral valve and area for rheumatism.

[Remarks]

The clinical manifestations of the disease are very complicated, and patients need to get plenty of rest and avoid tiredness. Critical patients with severe cardiac insufficiency or heart failure should be treated immediately with emergency drugs in an urgent attempt to save them.

III. Diseases of the Digestive System

1. Gastritis

[Pathogenesis and clinical manifestations]

This is an inflammatory disease of the gastric mucosa due to various causes. The onset of acute gastritis is sudden, and patients may suffer from pain or colic in the abdomen, nausea, vomiting and urgent watery diarrhea. Patients with severe acute gastritis may also have fever, dehydration and acidosis. Patients with chronic gastritis may suffer from epigastric distension, dull pain, belching, nausea, vomiting and poor appetite.

[Hand diagnosis]

In patients with acute gastritis, some nodules in a bright white color or in a red alternating with white are present in the stomach area. Dark red nodules in this area indicate congestion of mucosa of the stomach. In patients with chronic gastritis, some white spots are scattered over the stomach area. Yellow thickened skin similar to a callus in this area indicates chronic hypertrophic gastritis with chronic inflammation over a large area of gastric mucosa over a long time.

[Selection of points]

First-choice points: Point for pain of stomach and intestine and Wailaogong (EX-UE 8).

Secondary points: Stomach area and area of upper abdomen.

[Therapeutic methods]

Regular acupuncture is applied at the point for pain of stomach and intestine and Wàilaogong point, and massage or magnet therapy is performed in the stomach area and area of upper abdomen.

2. Peptic ulcer of stomach and duodenum

[Pathogenesis and clinical manifestation]

This is a disease involving ulcers in the stomach and duodenum caused by longstanding indigestion, extreme mental nervousness and dysfunction of the vegetative nervous system. Patients may suffer from regular epigastric pain, regurgitation of sour fluid, belching, nausea and vomiting.

[Hand diagnosis]

In patients with an ulcer in their stomach or duodenum, a dark red or blackish brown color may appears underneath the prominent skin over the stomach and duodenum areas. A blackish-brown color indicates that ulcers already have healed up. The presence of several white round patches alternating with some small fresh red spots in those areas indicates a possibility of bleeding over the ulcerated surface.

[Selection of points]

First-choice points: Point for pain of stomach and intestine and point of small intestine.

Secondary points: Wailaogong (EX-UE 8), stomach area and area of upper abdomen.

[Therapeutic methods]

Regular acupuncture is applied at the point for pain of stomach and intestine and point of small intestine, and massage is performed in the stomach area and area of upper abdomen and also at Wailaogong point.

[Remarks]

In patients with a peptic ulcer with early symptoms and signs of bleeding ulcers, their stool should be examined for blood to determine necessary treatment.

3. Acute enteritis

[Pathogenesis and clinical manifestations]

This is an acute inflammation of intestinal mucosa caused by eating and drinking too much at one meal or eating food contaminated by bacteria. Clinical symptoms include a sudden onset, frequent bowel movement, abdominal pain, vomiting, loose or watery stool, and even dehydration in the severe attacks.

[Hand diagnosis]

One or several red or dark red spots or patches are present in the area of upper, middle and lower abdomen and the blood congestion in a dark red color can be seen in the stomach area.

[Selection of points]

First-choice points: Hegu (LI 4), point for diarrhea and point of large intestine.

Secondary points: Area of abdomen.

[Therapeutic methods]

Regular acupuncture is applied at Hegu point, point for diarrhea and point of large intestine, and massage is performed in the area of abdomen.

4. Chronic colitis

[Pathogenesis and clinical manifestations]

The disease is also called chronic idiopathic ulcerative colitis with a superficial nonspecific inflammation of the colonic mucosa caused by immunological, mental and hereditary disturbances and nonspecific infection. Patients may suffer from diarrhea, abdominal pain, hematemesis, tenesmus [A painfully urgent but ineffectual attempt to urinate or defecate.], low fever, anemia and emaciation.

[Hand diagnosis]

One or several white or dark blue patches may appear in the region corresponding to the colon in the holographic area of lower abdomen. A red patch indicates severe abdominal pain and the presence of blood in the stool, and a dark red patch indicates resolution of the inflammation in colon.

[Selection of points]

First-choice points: Point of large intestine, point for diarrhea and Wailaogong (EX-UE 8).

Secondary points: Abdomen area and Shangyang (LI 1).

[Therapeutic methods]

Regular acupuncture is applied at the point of large intestine, point for diarrhea and Wailaogong point; bleeding therapy is applied at Shangyang point; and massage is performed in the abdomen area.

5. Constipation

[Pathogenesis and clinical manifestations]

Constipation usually is caused by mental and nervous disturbance, reduction of colonic tone, impairment of intestinal mucosa, and disappearance of the reflex to defecate. Besides difficult defecation of dry and hard stool and prolonged intervals between defecation of over 48 hours, patients also suffer from abdominal distension, headache, vertigo, poor appetite, nausea and insomnia.

[Hand diagnosis]

A diffuse red color with one or several deep red spots or patches may appear in the abdomen area.

[Selection of points]

First-choice points: Hegu (LI 4) and point of large intestine.

Secondary points: Wailaogong (EX-UE 8), point for pain of forehead and abdomen area.

[Therapeutic methods]

Regular acupuncture is applied at Hegu point, point of large intestine and Wailaogong point, and massage is performed at the point for pain of forehead and in the abdomen area.

[Remarks]

Acupuncture at Dachangshu (BL 52) and Baliao (BL 31-34) points can produce an excellent therapeutic effect to treat stubborn constipation.

6. Chronic cholecystitis

[Pathogenesis and clinical manifestations]

The disease is caused by an infection of intestinal bacteria, obstruction of the biliary tract and accumulation of bile. Patients may suffer from discomfort in the epigastric or right subcostal region, persistent dull pain, abdominal distension, nausea, belching, regurgitation of sour fluid and alternate voiding of dry and loose stool.

[Hand diagnosis]

One or several dull white or yellow spots or patches may be found in the gallbladder area. Sometimes, the spots are in a shape of grits with clear-cut margins to distinguish them from their surrounding skin.

[Selection of points]

First-choice points: Point of liver and point for pain of temple of head (migraine).

Secondary points: Gallbladder area and area of upper abdomen.

[Therapeutic methods]

Regular acupuncture is applied at the point for pain of temple of head; magnet therapy is applied on the gallbladder area; and massage is performed in the area of upper abdomen.

7. Hiccups

[Pathogenesis and clinical manifestations]

This spasm of the diaphragm muscle is caused by a spontaneous muscular contraction induced by the stimulation of the phrenic nerve. Hiccups may be caused by a cold, problems with the digestive organ or following an operation. Hiccups are also a clinical symptom of hysteria.

[Hand diagnosis]

A vertical long prominence of white shiny skin can be seen in the stomach area.

[Selection of points]

First-choice point: Point for hiccup.

Secondary point: Stomach area.

[Therapeutic methods]

Regular acupuncture is applied at bilateral points for hiccups, and massage is performed in the stomach area.

[Remarks]

Acupuncture may be applied at bilateral Neiguan (PC 6) points to relieve the stubborn hiccup.

8. Acid reflux

[Pathogenesis and clinical manifestations]

This is an inflammation of the lower segment of esophagus caused by a dysfunction of the cardioesophageal sphincter and the reflux of the contents of the stomach and duodenum. Patients with a mild type suffer from a burning sensation and pain behind the xiphoid process of the sternum, belching and vomiting. Patients with a severe type may suffer from dysphagia, bleeding, epigastric discomfort, poor appetite, indigestion and gradual loss of weight.

[Hand diagnosis]

In the early stages of the disease, some scattered white spots may appear in the esophagus area. The presence of some yellow nodules overlapping the white spots indicates a long clinical course of the disease. Spots in a red alternating with white or in a pure red color can show the seriousness of the disease.

[Selection of points]

First-choice points: Point for pain of stomach and intestine, Guanchong (SJ 1) and esophagus area.

Secondary points: Stomach area and area of upper abdomen.

[Therapeutic methods]

Regular acupuncture is applied at the point for pain of stomach and intestine and Guanchong point, and massage with thumb or magnet therapy is performed in the esophagus area, stomach area and area of upper abdomen.

9. Ptosis of stomach

[Pathogenesis and clinical manifestations]

This is a disease with a downward displacement of the stomach to an abnormally low level, even down to the pelvic cavity. Ptosis of the stomach can be divided into the congenital and acquired types. In patients of the former type with a congenital asthenic physique, the stomach is displaced downward along with almost all the other abdominal organs, such as the kidney. In the latter type, the stomach itself loses support from its surroundings due to reduced intraperitoneal pressure and flaccid abdominal walls. Patients may suffer from many digestive symptoms including abdominal distension, epigastric pain, poor appetite, vomiting and constipation.

[Hand diagnosis]

A white vertical elliptic patch or an elongate stripe is present in the basal region of the stomach area and near the kidney area.

[Selection of points]

First-choice points: Stomach area, point for pain of stomach and intestine and area of upper abdomen.

Secondary points: Wailaogong (EX-UE 8) and Hegu (LI 4) points.

[Therapeutic methods]

Regular acupuncture is applied at the point for pain of stomach and intestine, Wailaogong point and Hegu point and the massage or magnet therapy is performed in the stomach area and area of upper abdomen.

[Remarks]

During treatment, patients are asked to take frequent small meals and to lie down for a while after each meal. After each acupuncture treatment, patients are put into a Trendelenburg's position for 30 minutes.

10. Cholelithiasis (gallstone)

[Pathogenesis and clinical manifestation]

Gallstones may be present in the gallbladder, common bile duct and intrahepatic biliary ducts, and it is a problem closely related to infection of biliary ducts, stasis of bile and parasites in the biliary ducts. In early stages, the clinical manifestations may be nonspecific with patients complaining only of mild abdominal pain or indigestion. In acute stages, patients may suffer from severe epigastric pain, chills, fever, jaundice, nausea, vomiting and poor appetite.

[Hand diagnosis]

The presence of some hard nodules on the white bulging skin over the gallbladder area indicates a granular gallstone; and dark spots visible underneath white bulging skin in this area indicate a sandy gallstone. The presence of both hard nodules on the skin and dark spots beneath the skin indicates a mixture of granular and sandy gallstones.

[Selection of points]

First-choice points: Gallbladder area, area of upper abdomen and point for pain of temple of head.

Secondary points: Point of liver and Wailaogong (EX-UE 8).

[Therapeutic methods]

Regular acupuncture is applied at the point for pain of temple of head, point of liver and Wailaogong point, and thumb massage is performed in the gallbladder area and area of upper abdomen.

[Remarks]

An attack accompanied by severe epigastric pain, fever and jaundice indicates gallstones are obstructing the common bile duct. These patients should be treated immediately with antibiotics, spasmolytic drugs and even surgical intervention, if necessary.

IV. Diseases of the Endocrine System

1. Diabetes mellitus

[Pathogenesis and clinical manifestations]

This is a common endocrine disease with metabolic disorders of carbohydrate, fat, protein, water and electrolytes due to an absolute or relative deficiency of insulin. In early stages, patients may be free of pain. Its typical symptoms are the so-called "three increases and one decrease," namely the increase of urination, water drinking and food intake and the decrease of body weight with complications of ketoacidosis, infections, arteriosclerosis, lesions of the capillary blood vessels in the kidney and retina of eye, and peripheral neuritis.

[Hand diagnosis]

The holographic area of diabetes mellitus is below the area of vermiform appendix on the hypothenar prominence of palm. The findings of hand diagnosis of this disease are varied with its clinical manifestations. Dark yellow, white and red in this area indicate an increase of urination, water drinking and food intake respectively. The presence of some dark yellow or dark brown spots in the bladder area indicates a retention of urine caused by diabetes mellitus.

[Selection of points]

First-choice points: Point of lung, point of spleen and point of kidney.

Secondary points: Lung area, spleen area, pancreas area, kidney area and bladder area.

[Therapeutic methods]

Regular acupuncture is applied at the points of lung, spleen and kidney; massage is performed in the lung, spleen, kidney and pancreas areas. Massage also may be performed in the bladder area, if a patient develops retention of urine.

[Remarks]

This treatment is applicable to diabetes mellitus of type II. However, patients of insulin-dependent type should be treated with drugs to control hyperglycemia.

2. Menopausal syndrome

[Pathogenesis and clinical manifestations]

The disease usually afflicts women 45-55 years old with impaired ovarian functions around menopause, although it may be due to other causes. As demonstrated in clinical studies in recent years, menopausal syndrome may also attack males with reduced reproductive functions. The common clinical symptoms of the disease are sadness, anxiety, fear, insomnia, headache, vertigo, poor mental concentration, unstable blood pressure, profuse sweating, edema, abnormal skin sensations, and irregular menses in women.

[Hand diagnosis]

In patients suffering the disease, a red color may appear in the heart area, usually in the area of right heart and sometimes the red color can be seen throughout the whole thenar prominence. In addition, several white thickened spots are present in the uterus area and some abnormal findings can also be seen in the head area, area for insomnia and area for fatigue.

[Selection of points]

First-choice points: Heart area and area of reproductive organs.

Secondary points: Head area and areas for insomnia, fatigue, hypertension and hypotension.

[Therapeutic methods]

This is a chronic syndrome, therefore, an important treatment is massage applied at all points and areas mentioned above. As a supplemental therapy, psychotherapy and a regular life-style is also useful in achieving a good therapeutic effect.

[Remarks]

For patients with severe symptoms, a combination of psychotherapy, Western drugs or Chinese herbs should be prescribed.

V. Diseases of the Urogenital System

1. Urinary tract infections

[Pathogenesis and clinical manifestations]

This is an inflammatory disease of urinary system organs caused by bacteria directly invading the urinary tract. It can be divided into upper (pyelonephritis) and lower (cystitis) urinary tract infections as well as acute and chronic infections. The disease usually attacks women of 20-40 years old. Patients may suffer from urgent and painful urination in acute urethritis; distension and pain in lower abdomen and tenderness in the bladder region in acute cystitis; and chills, high fever, lumbago and a throbbing pain in the kidney region in acute pyelonephritis.

[Hand diagnosis]

In the bladder area, the prominent skin in white or a red alternating with white indicates chronic cystitis. A red or pink color in the whole bladder area indicates acute cystitis. A dark purple in the kidney area indicates pyelonephritis.

[Selection of points]

First-choice points: Point for frequent urination and point of kidney.

Secondary points: Bladder area, kidney area and waist area.

[Therapeutic methods]

Regular acupuncture is applied at the point for frequent urination and point of kidney, and massage is performed in the bladder, kidney and waist areas.

2. Retention of urine

[Pathogenesis and clinical manifestations]

This is a disorder of usual ability to discharge urine with distension of lower abdomen, but the disorder is not caused by an organic obstruction in the urinary tract.

[Hand diagnosis]

A dark red or light brown patch is present in the bladder area.

[Selection of points]

First-choice points: Point of Sanjiao and point of kidney.

Secondary point: Bladder area.

[Therapeutic methods]

Regular acupuncture is applied at the point of Sanjiao and point of kidney, and massage is performed in the bladder area.

3. Vesical stone

[Pathogenesis and clinical manifestations]

A stone in the bladder may produce local trauma, obstruction and infection in the bladder and cause difficult and painful urination and terminal hematuria. It is more common in young boys and old men.

[Hand diagnosis]

In the bladder area, the presence of granular spots indicates the small vesical stones, but the presence of a white round papule indicates a large stone. Yellow spots indicate a long clinical course of the disease.

[Selection of points]

First-choice points: Point of kidney and bladder area.

Secondary point: Point of Sanjiao.

[Therapeutic methods]

Regular acupuncture is applied at the point of Sanjiao and point of kidney, and massage is performed in the bladder area, three to five times per day according to the severity of disease.

4. Kidney and ureter stone

[Pathogenesis and clinical manifestations]

A kidney and ureter stone may cause obstruction in the upper, middle or lower segment of ureter, trauma, infection and retention of urine. Patients may suffer from hematuria and renal colic with radiating pain in the back and along the pathway of ureter. Kidney and ureter stones usually are a problem among youths 20-50 years in age, and it is more common in men than in women.

[Hand diagnosis]

One or several dark red or shiny irregular nodules similar to grits are present in the kidney area, and gravely irregular nodules surrounded by a white or red halo can be seen in the ureter area (between the kidney area and bladder area).

[Selection of points]

First-choice points: Point of Sanjiao, point of kidney and ureter area.

Secondary point: Kidney area and back area.

[Therapeutic methods]

Regular acupuncture is applied at the point of Sanjiao and point of kidney, and massage is performed in the ureter, kidney and back areas.

5. Prostatitis

[Pathogenesis and clinical manifestations]

As a disease secondary to urethritis and other inflammations of the body, prostatitis usually attacks young men. In acute prostatitis, patients may suffer from high fever, chills, frequent and urgent urination. Chronic patients may suffer from lumbago, discomfort in the perineum, spermatic cord and testis, slightly increased frequency of urination, incomplete voiding of urine, and discharge of white mucus from the urethra.

[Hand diagnosis]

In early stages, one or several pale shiny nodules are sparsely scattered in the area of prostate gland, but they become dense in patients with severe infection of the gland. In chronic patients, one or several yellow round nodules can be found in this area.

[Selection of points]

First-choice points: Area of reproductive organs and point of Mingmen.

Secondary point: Kidney area.

[Therapeutic methods]

Regular acupuncture is applied at the point of Mingmen, and massage is performed in the kidney area and area of reproductive organs.

6. Chronic glomerulonephritis (Bright's disease)

[Pathogenesis and clinical manifestations]

This is a disease involving inflammatory damage to the renal capillaries. Its pathogenic causes are still unknown, but according to clinical observations, the disease in 85 percent of patients is related to an infection of hemolytic streptococcus. The clinical course of the disease is very long, and patients may have protein in their urine, microscopic hematuria, edema, hypertension, abdominal distension, diarrhea, soreness and pain in waist and leg, an intolerance of cold and cold limbs.

[Hand diagnosis]

One or several spots in a red alternating with white color or a few light-yellow nodules can be seen in the kidney area of one or both sides. In patients with edema, a white patch can be found in the area for edema. A dark red or dark gray color is present in the area for hypertension in patients with hypertension.

[Selection of points]

First-choice points: Kidney area, point of kidney and point for lumbago.

Secondary points: Area for edema and area for hypertension.

[Therapeutic methods]

Regular acupuncture is applied at the point of kidney and point for lumbago, and massage is performed in the kidney area, area for edema and area for hypertension.

[Remarks]

This is a chronic disease with a prolonged clinical course, so it needs persistent treatment. A combined therapy of Western medicine and Traditional Chinese Medicine is indicated in patients with renal failure.

7. Chronic pyelonephritis

[Pathogenesis and clinical manifestations]

This is a chronic infection of the renal pelvis and parenchyma of one or both kidneys caused by a direct invasion of nonspecific bacteria through regional, retrograde, blood borne or lymphatic transmission. The chronic pyelonephritis is derived from acute pyelonephritis and the incidence of the disease is higher in women. Patients may suffer from lumbago, tiredness, irregular low fever, mild edema, and increased frequency of urination at night.

[Hand diagnosis]

One or several dark red or bright white spots may appear in the kidney area on one or both sides. In patients with edema, a white patch can be found in the area for edema and in patients with lumbago, one or several white or light yellow spots may appear in the area for lumbago.

[Selection of points]

First-choice points: Kidney area, point of kidney and waist area.

Secondary points: Area for edema and point for lumbago.

[Therapeutic methods]

Regular acupuncture is applied at the point of kidney and point for lumbago; massage is performed in the kidney area, waist area and area for edema; and the magnetic plates are applied in the kidney and waist areas.

[Remarks]

Patients should take care of their personal hygiene to prevent retrograde infection or urinary tract infection, avoid overfatigue, reduce sexual activity, drink more water and avoid spicy foods. For very sick patients, other therapies should be adopted in combination with this treatment.

VI. Diseases of the Nervous System

1. Neurasthenia

[Pathogenesis and clinical manifestation]

This is a common neurotic disease characterized by high excitability and rapid fatigue caused by poor adjustment between excitation and depression in the cerebral cortex after mental trauma or a longstanding nervous disorder. The clinical manifestations of the disease include dizziness, tinnitus, a heavy feeling in the head, vertigo, poor memory, heart palpitations, profuse sweating, reduced sexual desire, and irregular menses. Patients may also suffer from lethargy, drowsiness and tiredness in the day and insomnia, excitation and dreaminess at night.

[Hand diagnosis]

Neurasthenia is a complicated disease with multiple organs involved, therefore, the findings of hand diagnosis are very much varied. In general, red patches or alternating with white color can be seen in the head area. Red or dark red patches can be found in the area for dizziness. White papules or alternating with white color can be seen in the area for insomnia and — if the insomnia is very severe — the skin over this area is bright white in color. A red alternating with white color in the area for fatigue indicates general weakness and sleeplessness. A red color in the heart area (even in the whole thenar prominence) indicates heart palpitations and profuse sweating due to excessiveness of heart fire. A pure white color or alternating with red color in the area for dreaminess indicates patients susceptible to insomnia.

[Selection of points]

First-choice points: Hegu (LI 4), Zhongchong (PC 9), Laogong (PC 8), area for dizziness and area for insomnia.

Secondary points: Heart area, area for dreaminess and head area.

[Therapeutic methods]

Regular acupuncture is applied at Hegu, Zhongchong and Laogong points; bleeding therapy is applied at Zhongchong point; and massage is performed in the heart area and areas for dizziness, insomnia and dreaminess.

2. Trigeminal neuralgia

[Pathogenesis and clinical manifestations]

The cause of the disease is still unknown, but it may be induced by an inflammation of eye, nose and teeth, pressure of tumors against a nerve or poor nourishment of a nerve. Patients may suffer from paroxysmal attacks of severe lightning pain with sensations of being cut, pricked or burned. Each attack may last for a few seconds or minutes and several attacks or a few dozens of attacks may flare up per day. At the same time, the involved side during the severe attacks may exhibit facial convulsions, a shedding of tears and a runny nose. This desease usually attacks people at the age of 40-60. It is more common in women than men.

[Hand diagnosis]

In the early stage, one or several white spots are present on the proximal crease of middle finger in the head area. In chronic patients, one or several purplish red, blue or yellow patches can be seen in the head area and a white color is present in the eye area.

[Selection of points]

First-choice points: Hegu (LI 4), Shangyang (LI 1), point for pain of eye and point for pain of forehead.

Secondary points: Head area and eye area.

[Therapeutic methods]

Regular acupuncture is applied at Hegu and Shangyang points, point for pain of eye and point for pain of forehead, and massage is performed in the head and eye areas.

3. Vascular headache

[Pathogenesis and clinical manifestations]

This is a medical name for migraine, for which the cause is unknown. Its important clinical symptom is the unilateral, throbbing and distending headache over the vertex, occiput and orbit regions of head, accompanied with nausea, vomiting, shedding of tears and vertigo for several dozens of minutes and even a few days. Attacks of migraine may be induced by mental nervousness, emotional disturbance, tiredness and attack of wind. Its incidence is higher in young women than that in men.

[Hand diagnosis]

The presence of white patches in the left or right side of the basal crease of middle finger indicates migraine of the left or right head respectively.

[Selection of points]

First-choice points: Point for migraine and Hegu (LI 4).

Secondary points: Head area and eye area.

[Therapeutic methods]

Regular acupuncture is applied at the point for migraine and Hegu point, and massage is performed in the head area and eye area.

4. Sequelae of stroke

[Pathogenesis and clinical manifestations]

This is an acute disease in patients above middle age and it can be divided into the hemorrhagic and ischemic type. Cerebral hemorrhage and subarachnoid hemorrhage are classified in the former group; and cerebral thrombosis and cerebral embolism are classified in the latter group. Patients may suffer from a sudden loss of consciousness, coma, aphasia and sensory and motor disturbance on one side of the body. The results of a stroke — including hemiplegia, central facial paralysis and aphasia — are indications of this therapy.

[Hand diagnosis]

The presence of a gray or grayish blue patch in the corresponding region of the head area indicates patients in the recovery stage of a stroke (with sequelae).

[Selection of points]

First-choice points: Hegu (LI 4), head area, Yangxi (LI 5) and Houxi (SI 3).

Secondary points: Eye area, cheek area and Zhongzhu (LR 6).

[Therapeutic methods]

Regular acupuncture is applied at Hegu, Yangxi and Houxi points, and massage is performed in the head area. Massage is again performed in the eye and cheek areas for patients with deviation of eye and mouth, and acupuncture is applied at Zhongzhu point for patients with paralysis of an upper limb.

[Remarks]

In the early stage following a stroke, hand acupuncture therapy can produce a good therapeutic effect. The body acupuncture and massage of the whole body to promote blood circulation and enhance recovery of nervous tissues are necessary to treat patients with severe sequelae of stroke.

5. Sequelae of brain injury

[Pathogenesis and clinical manifestations]

The sequelae of brain injury include retrograde amnesia (poor memory), headache, dizziness, nausea, vomiting and drowsiness after a brain injury accompanied by a temporary loss of consciousness. In some patients, a distending and throbbing headache exacerbated after manual labor, dizziness, vertigo, tinnitus, poor memory and insomnia may persist for more than three months.

[Hand diagnosis]

A blue or bluish purple patches with engorged subcutaneous capillary blood vessels are present in the head area. In patients with dizziness, insomnia and poor memory, dark purple patches may appear in the area for dizziness and some spots in a red alternating with white color are present in the area for insomnia.

[Selection of points]

First-choice points: Point for pain of forehead, point for pain of vertex of head and point for pain of occiput of head.

Secondary points: Head area, area for dizziness, area for insomnia and Zhongchong (PC 9).

[Therapeutic methods]

Regular acupuncture is applied at points for pain of forehead, vertex of head and occiput of head; bleeding therapy is applied at Zhongchong point; and massage is performed in the head area and areas for dizziness and insomnia.

6. Neuralgia sciatica

[Pathogenesis and clinical manifestations]

This is a disease more common in men of middle age. Its symptoms can include pain in areas that are on the passage and in the innervating region of the sciatic nerve — the buttocks, posterior side of the thigh and the lateral aspect of the leg and foot. The disease can be divided into a primary and secondary type. Primary neuralgia sciatica with a lesion of the nerve itself is caused by infection and induced by an attack of coldness. The secondary type is caused by pressure applied to the nerve by its neighboring structures, such as the herniation of the lumbar intervertebral disc, tumors, inflammation of piriform muscle, and sacroiliac arthritis.

[Hand diagnosis]

A white papule in the waist area indicates neuralgia sciatica with radiating pain to the waist and leg caused by the herniation of lumbar intervertebral disc. The presence of a bluish purple or blue patch in the area of lumbar and sacrum spine on the back of the hand indicates neuralgia sciatica caused by an inflammation of the piriform muscle or sacroiliac arthritis.

[Selection of points]

First-choice points: Point for neuralgia sciatica and point for lumbago.

Secondary points: Waist area, liver area and area of lumbar and sacral spine.

[Therapeutic methods]

Regular acupuncture is applied at the point for neuralgia sciatica and point for lumbago, and massage is performed in the waist area, liver area and area of lumbar and sacral spine.

7. Facial palsy

[Pathogenesis and clinical manifestations]

This is a syndrome with inflammation of the facial nerve caused by trauma or local infection. Therefore, it is a peripheral type of facial palsy. Patients may show shallow or flattened forehead wrinkles, leakage of air from the mouth in a cheek-blowing test, a shallow nasolabial groove of involved side, a widened palpebral fissure, shedding of tears, photophobia (fear of light) and impairment of cheek movement.

[Hand diagnosis]

One or several pink or dark red spots or patches are present in the cheek area and some pink spots appear in the eye area.

[Selection of points]

First-choice points: Hegu (LI 4), Zhongzhu (SJ 3), point for pain of eye, and cheek area.

Secondary points: Head area and nose area.

[Therapeutic methods]

Regular acupuncture is applied at Hegu and Zhongzhu points and point for pain of eye and massage is performed in the cheek, head and nose areas.

8. Facial spasm

[Pathogenesis and clinical manifestations]

This is a disease with irregular paroxysmal attacks of spontaneous convulsions of the facial muscles. In the early stage, the orbicular muscle of the eye is first involved in intermittent spasms of the eyelid and then other facial muscles of the same side are affected in succession. The cause of the disease is still unknown, but it may be induced by fatigue and mental stress.

[Hand diagnosis]

One or several dark gray or brown spots or patches can be seen in the cheek area, and yellowish brown nodules indicate a disease with a long clinical course.

[Selection of points]

First-choice points: Zhongzhu (SJ 3), Hegu (LI 4) and cheek area.

Secondary points: Eye area, nose area and mouth area.

[Therapeutic methods]

Regular acupuncture is applied at Zhongzhu and Hegu points, and massage is performed in the eye, nose and mouth areas.

9. Neuralgia of the greater occipital nerve

[Pathogenesis and clinical manifestations]

This is a disease with a paroxysmal or continuous pain in the innervating area of the greater occipital nerve on one or both sides, radiating to the vertex of head. It is mainly induced by an attack of coldness, soft tissue injury of head and neck, sneezing or cough. In general, its prognosis is good.

[Hand diagnosis]

Some white or dark red spots are visible in the head area, and small blue engorged blood vessels may be present in the area of occiput of head.

[Selection of points]

First-choice points: Hegu (LI 4), head area and area of occiput of head.

Secondary points: Point for pain of occiput of head and point for pain of vertex of head.

[Therapeutic methods]

Regular acupuncture is applied at Hegu, point for pain of occiput of head and point for pain of vertex of head; bleeding therapy is applied to squeeze 2-3 drops of blood from each of the points for pain of both occiput and vertex of head; and massage is performed in the head area and area of occiput of head.

[Remarks]

Hand acupuncture therapy can produce a good effect to control an attack of this neuralgia. If the treatment can be started in the early stage of the disease, an excellent result can be achieved. Patients should avoid spicy food.

10. Senile dementia

[Pathogenesis and clinical manifestations]

This is a chronic progressive disease of elderly people with specific pathological changes in the brain tissues due to infection, intoxication and some mental factors. Because of the diffuse atrophy and degeneration of the brain, patients suffer a gradual loss of memory and impairment of intelligence — important clinical manifestations of the disease. As the earliest symptom, the change of personality is characterized by selfishness, subjectivity, stubbornness and poor concentration. This is followed by a decline of memory and judgement. Patients may become highly irritable and indulge in destructive behavior because of suspicions and hallucinations. In the late stage, patients may stay in bed all day long with urination and defecation out of control. Following the aging process, they may develop gray hair, loss of teeth, atrophy of the skin, tremor of hand and tongue, and visual and auditory impairment.

[Hand diagnosis]

In this disease, the findings of hand diagnosis are very complicated, but one or several dark blue or dark gray patches can often be seen in the head area and some small prominent bluish purple blood vessels can be found underneath the skin in this area.

[Selection of points]

First-choice points: Head area, Houxi (SI 3) and Zhongchong (PC 9).

Secondary points: Hegu (LI 4), kidney area, area for dizziness and eye area.

[Therapeutic methods]

Regular acupuncture is applied at Hegu and Houxi points; the three-edged needle is used to prick Zhongchong point for bleeding of 2-3 drops of blood; and massage is performed in the head and kidney areas and area for dizziness.

[Remarks]

Besides hand acupuncture therapy, other Western drugs and Chinese herbs also should be administered to treat patients of the disease.

11. Spasm of diaphragmatic muscles

[Pathogenesis and clinical manifestations]

This is a common symptom with automatic and intermittent contractions and spasms of the diaphragmatic muscles from stimulation produced by many causes to the diaphragm center in the medulla oblongata. Inhalation of cold air, mental factors and chronic diseases of the stomach and intestine may induce attacks of diaphragmatic spasm. In mild instances, the attack may spontaneously stop without any treatment, but in severe cases, the attack may last days and nights or relapse over several dozens of days and every few months.

[Hand diagnosis]

One or several white or bluish white patches may appear in the upper region of stomach area and a vertical white cord can be found in the upper and middle regions of stomach area.

[Selection of points]

First-choice points: Stomach area, point of Sanjiao and esophagus area.

Secondary point: Shixuan (EX-UE 11).

[Therapeutic methods]

Regular acupuncture is applied at the point of Sanjiao; bleeding therapy with a three-edged needle is applied at Shixuan points; and massage with thumb is performed in the stomach and esophagus areas.

VII. Infectious Diseases

1. Influenza

[Pathogenesis and clinical manifestations]

This is an acute viral infection of upper respiratory tract. The disease can be divided into common cold and epidemic influenza, and it may be transmitted through all four seasons. Patients may suffer from headache, fever, chills, weakness, aching of limbs, nasal obstruction, runny nose, sore throat and cough.

[Hand diagnosis]

One or several white spots or patches are found in the head area. Superficial spots in a pale white color or a red alternating with white color are present in the nose area. Similar findings of hand diagnosis also can be seen in the throat area.

[Selection of points]

First-choice points: Hegu (LI 4), Yuji (LU 10), point for pain of forehead and point of throat.

Secondary points: Point of lung, point for high fever, nose area and throat area.

[Therapeutic methods]

Regular acupuncture is applied at Hegu, Yuji, point for pain of forehead and point of throat. It also may be applied at the point for high fever in patients with high fever and at the point of lung in patients with cough. Massage is performed in the nose and throat areas.

2. German measles

[Pathogenesis and clinical manifestations]

This is an eruptive epidemic disease caused by rubella virus with a name of "Fengsha" (wind rashes) in Traditional Chinese Medicine. It is transmitted in the spring and autumn among children below 5 years of age. Patients usually have a contact history 2-3 weeks before the onset of disease, 1-2 days later, skin rashes may appear on the face and trunk, and then the rashes may spread all over the body in one day. Patients may also suffer from fever, cough and sore throat. Together with the relief of symptoms, the skin rashes may disappear in 2-3 days without pigmentation and peeling of the skin.

[Hand diagnosis]

Some white spots, patches or papules may appear in the skin area and the white spots are also present in the throat area and trachea area.

[Selection of points]

First-choice points: Yuji (LU 10), Shangyang (LI 1), Yemen (SJ 2) and point of lung.

Secondary points: Skin area, trachea area and throat area.

[Therapeutic methods]

Regular acupuncture is applied at Yuji and Yemen points; bleeding therapy is applied at Shangyang and point of lung; and massage is performed in the skin, trachea and throat areas.

3. Whooping cough

[Pathogenesis and clinical manifestations]

This is a common infectious disease of respiratory tract in children and it is caused by Bordetella pertussis. The clinical symptoms in the early stage are similar to those of the common cold, but the cough is gradually worse and particularly serious at night. Following each paroxysmal attack of short spastic cough from more than 10 to few dozens times, patients always produce a whooping noise of high pitch due to spasm of the glottis. Patients may also suffer from vomiting, an ulcer of the frenulum of the tongue, swelling of eyelids, subconjunctival hemorrhage and nasal bleeding.

[Hand diagnosis]

Some pale white spots are sparsely scattered in the nose, throat, trachea and bronchus areas.

[Selection of points]

First-choice points: Shaoshang (LU 11), Yuji (LU 10) and point of lung.

Secondary points: Trachea area, bronchus area and nose area.

[Therapeutic methods]

Regular acupuncture is applied at Shaoshang, Yuji and point of lung and massage is performed in the trachea, bronchus and nose areas.

4. Pulmonary tuberculosis

[Pathogenesis and clinical manifestations]

This is a chronic consumptive disease of the lung caused by Mycobacterium tuberculosis. It is an air borne infectious disease of the respiratory tract, transmitted through contact with communicable patients, but the communication of disease depends on the body resistance of individuals and the violence of the tuberculous bacilli. Pulmonary tuberculosis is usually a chronic disease, but the onset of the disease may be sudden in some patients. Coughing and expectoration of blood or of blood-streaked sputum (hemoptysis) are the common symptoms involving the respiratory tract. A low fever, night sweating and weakness are the common general symptoms.

[Hand diagnosis]

The skin in the trachea area is red in color. Some small dark hard nodules in the left (right) lung area indicate the calcified foci of tuberculous lesions in the corresponding lung. The presence of one or a few round or elliptic spot indicate pulmonary tuberculosis in the early stage. If the spots are in gray color or a mixed color of red and white, the disease is in the active stage. Fresh red spots similar to blood that has oozed from pin holes in the skin in the lung area indicate hemoptysis.

[Selection of points]

First-choice points: Yuji (LU 10), Laogong (PC 8), lung point and Shaoshang (LU 11).

Secondary points: Lung area, trachea area and area for deficiency of qi.

[Therapeutic methods]

Regular acupuncture is applied at Yuji, Laogong and point of lung; bleeding therapy is applied at Shaoshang point; and massage is performed in the lung and trachea areas and area for deficiency of qi.

[Remarks]

Chemicals appropriate for the treatment of tuberculosis should be prescribed to patients with typical symptoms and signs of active pulmonary tuberculosis.

5. Viral hepatitis

[Pathogenesis and clinical manifestations]

This is an infectious disease of the digestive tract caused by hepatitis virus with symptoms of poor appetite, nausea, epigastric discomfort, pain in the liver region and weakness. Fever and jaundice may appear in some patients. If the disease is not treated properly and the clinical course lasts over a prolonged period, viral hepatitis can turn into chronic hepatitis. Hepatitis A is transmitted by contaminated food and drink. Therefore, an epidemic of the disease may break out if patients carrying the disease can not be adequately isolated. Hepatitis B and non-A non-B hepatitis are blood borne infectious diseases transmitted through contaminated blood products and instruments for injection.

[Hand diagnosis]

In the liver area, some densely assembled spots in a red alternating with white color can be seen in patients of acute hepatitis; and the dark red and dark purple spots are also visible in this area of chronic patients.

[Selection of points]

First-choice points: Point of liver, point for pain of temple of head and point of spleen.

Secondary points: Liver area, stomach area and abdomen area.

[Therapeutic methods]

Regular acupuncture is applied at the point of liver, point for pain of temple of head and point of spleen, and massage is performed in the liver, stomach and spleen areas.

[Remarks]

Patients with viral hepatitis should take total bed rest and a high carbohydrate, high protein and low fat diet.

6. Bacillary dysentery

[Pathogenesis and clinical manifestations]

This is an enteric infectious disease caused by Bacillus dysenteriae with a diffuse inflammation in the colon. The disease can be divided into the acute and chronic types. Patients may suffer from abdominal pain, fever, chills, nausea, vomiting, poor appetite, a painfully urgent but ineffectual attempt to urinate or defecate, and diarrhea with discharge of pus and blood in stool for several dozens times per day.

[Hand diagnosis]

A vertical long patch in a white color or a red alternating with white color on the left side of the area of lower abdomen (near the left lower part of the hypothenar prominence) indicates acute bacillary dysentery. A patch in a red alternating with white color covering the whole area of lower abdomen indicates fulminating toxic dysentery.

[Selection of points]

First-choice points: Hegu (LI 4), point of large intestine and point of Sanjiao.

Secondary points: Zhongchong (PC 9), point for high fever and area of lower abdomen.

[Therapeutic methods]

Regular acupuncture is applied at Hegu point, point of large intestine, point of Sanjiao and point for high fever; bleeding therapy is applied at Zhongchong point; and massage is performed in the area of lower abdomen.

7. Malaria

[Pathogenesis and clinical manifestations]

· This is a parasitic disease in human beings caused by plasmodia and transmitted by mosquitoes. Malaria epidemics usually burst out in the summer and autumn, and patients often have a resident history in the epidemic region. Patients always suffer from regular attacks of intermittent chills, high fever and sweating. In pernicious malaria, the attack comes once a day and lasts for 6-10 hours or longer; in tertian malaria, the attack comes in an interval of every 48 hrs; and in quartan malaria, the attack comes in an interval of every 72 hrs. Patients suffer from no symptoms in the period between the two successive attacks, but they may show clinical manifestations of anemia and an enlarged spleen in late stages.

[Hand diagnosis]

The presence of a yellow, yellowish brown (callus color) or a light brown papule in the spleen area indicates an enlarged spleen.

The presence of one or several patches in a red alternating with white color or in a dark purple color in the liver area indicates the invasion of plasmodia into the liver.

[Selection of points]

First-choice points: Point for malaria, Laogong (PC 8), Houxi (SI 3) and Yemen (SJ 2) points.

Secondary points: Point of liver, point of spleen, liver area, spleen area and Baxie (EX-UE 9) points.

[Therapeutic methods]

Regular acupuncture is applied at the point for malaria, Laogong, Houxi, Yemen, point of liver and point of spleen; bleeding therapy is applied at Baxie points; and massage is performed in the liver and spleen areas.

[Remarks]

Antimalarial drugs, such as chloroquine and injection of arteannuin should be prescribed to patients of malaria, because patients of the disease usually have a sudden onset, violent clinical course and poor prognosis.

Section 2 Common Disorders Related to Surgery and Orthopedics

1. Postoperative abdominal distension

[Pathogenesis and clinical manifestations]

This is a postoperative complication of temporary intestinal paralysis as an after-effect of a surgery. The clinical symptoms are abdominal distension, lack of appetite, nausea, no gas or feces discharged from the intestine, and a reduction or elimination of any intestinal gurgling sound. Patients may also suffer from shortness of breath and dyspnea due to abdominal distension and an elevation of the diaphragm. Symptoms may come on and last from the 2nd to 5th postoperative day.

[Hand diagnosis]

The whole abdomen area is bulging and in a red alternating with white color.

[Selection of points]

First-choice points: Hegu (LI 4), point of large intestine and point of small intestine.

Secondary point: Abdomen area.

[Therapeutic methods]

Regular acupuncture is applied at Hegu, point of large intestine and point of small intestine, and massage is performed in the abdomen area.

2. Hyperplasia of breast

[Pathogenesis and clinical manifestations]

This is a benign hyperplasia of the interstitial tissues of breast, including the hyperplasia of tissues around the glandular dusts, hyperplasia of papillary endothelium in the glandular ducts, and hyperplasia of lobular substantial tissues. It is a common disease of women between 25-40 years in age. The hyperplastic masses may be located in one or both breasts, and their size can vary with the emotional disturbance and the cyclic change of menses. The pathogenesis of the disease is related to an endocrine disturbance and dysfunction of the ovary.

[Hand diagnosis]

Some small white spots in the left and/or right chest (lung) areas indicate hyperplasia of breast with pain in the early stage. A brown callus-like hard papule in this area indicates hyperplasia of the breast with a long clinical course. The bluish-white patch indicates severe pain in the corresponding region of the breast. The severity of pain is in proportion with the darkness of the blue color.

[Selection of points]

First-choice points: Shaoze (SI 1), Shaochong (HT 9) and point for pain of chest.

Secondary points: Left (right) area of chest and lung, upper portion of area of reproductive organs and liver area.

[Therapeutic methods]

Regular acupuncture is applied at Shaoze, Shaochong and point for pain of chest; the bleeding therapy is applied at Shaoze point for patients with severe pain; and massage is performed in the left (right) area of chest and lung, upper portion of the area of reproductive organs and liver area.

3. Hemorrhoids

[Pathogenesis and clinical manifestations]

Important symptoms of this common anal disease include hemorrhage, prolapse of hemorrhoids, constipation, and local swelling, itching and pain. According to the location of hemorrhoids, the disease can be divided into internal, external and mixed hemorrhoids. Hemorrhoids often are caused by always taking the same sitting posture, overfatigue, drinking too much alcohol and eating too much spicy food, habitual constipation, chronic diarrhea or dysentery, and pregnancy.

[Hand diagnosis]

Some dark blue nodules in the anus area indicate hemorrhoids. In patients with local pain, marked swelling and less hemorrhaging, the nodules are white in color. The nodules in a red color or a red alternating with white color are present in this area of patients with severe hemorrhage. Dry yellow nodules in this area indicate the healed hemorrhoids.

[Selection of points]

First-choice points: Shangyang (LI 1), Hegu (LI 4) and Laogong (PC 8).

Secondary points: Anus area and rectum area.

[Therapeutic methods]

Regular acupuncture is applied at Hegu and Laogong points; bleeding therapy is applied at Shangyang point and in the anus area; and massage is performed in the rectum area.

4. Acute lumbar sprain

[Pathogenesis and clinical manifestations]

This is a sudden injury of the soft tissues in the lumbar region with lumbago and a limitation of movement in the waist as its important symptoms. The injury usually is produced by lifting or carrying a heavy burden in an awkward posture, inadequate physical exertion or falling down. Because of severe lumbago, patients may typically exhibit a rigid board-like back that makes it difficult to bend forward or backward, to exert strength with the waist and to walk. A tender spot can be detected at the transverse process in the injured region.

[Hand diagnosis]

A dominant red color alternating with a white color in a location of the waist area indicates lumbago caused by the trauma or acute sprain in the corresponding region of the lower back.

[Selection of points]

First-choice point: Point for lumbago.

Secondary point: Waist area.

[Therapeutic methods]

Regular acupuncture is applied at the point for lumbago, and massage is performed in the waist area. At the same time, patients are asked to move their waists. The lumbago may be relieved following one to two treatments.

5. Stiff neck

[Pathogenesis and clinical manifestations]

This is a simple acute attack of neck muscles with rigidity, aching and limitation of movement of the neck, caused by inadequate pillows, improper sleeping posture or an attack of wind and coldness in all four seasons. In general, stiffness and aching of the neck may suddenly be felt by patients in the morning after they get up and try to move their neck. The movement of neck is limited and some tender spots can be easily detected in the involved muscles. The symptoms can be reduced or temporarily relieved by a hot compress. This mild type of disease may be spontaneously cured in 3-5 days, but a severe attack with pain radiating to the head and arm may last for several weeks.

[Hand diagnosis]

In the hand diagnosis, the corresponding location of Dazhui (DU 21) point on the body lies on the dorsal side of the metacarpophalangeal joint of middle finger. The appearance of a brown or brownish black color in a defined region of Dazhui area indicates the corresponding location of the involved neck muscles causing a stiff neck.

[Selection of points]

First-choice points: Point for pain of neck and point for stiff neck.

Secondary points: Houxi (SI 3) and Qiangu (SI 2).

[Therapeutic methods]

Regular acupuncture is applied at the point for pain of neck, point for stiff neck, Houxi and Qiangu points. Patients are asked to move their neck during the treatment. The suffering will be relieved completely after one-two treatments.

6. Cervical spondylosis

[Pathogenesis and clinical manifestations]

The disease is also called cervical syndrome involving a group of symptoms caused by stimulation or pressure applied to the blood vessels, nerves and spinal cord of the neck. What is produced is the loss of normal cervical spinal curvature, mechanical imbalance in the skeletal system of neck and degeneration of intervertebral discs, joints and ligaments of the cervical spinal column. Pathological changes primarily are caused by external trauma, chronic strain of soft tissues and attack of wind, cold and dampness pathogens. The important symptoms of the disease are neck pain, shoulder and arm pain, numbness in the arm, limitation of the movement of the neck, vertigo, nausea, vomiting, tinnitus, deafness, blurred vision and even a limitation of movement or paralysis of the upper and lower limbs.

[Hand diagnosis]

In the corresponding location of the cervical spine in the area of the spinal column, one to three dark papules or one dark yellow or yellowish brown pigmented patch (similar to a senile patch) can be found in patients of this disease.

[Selection of points]

First-choice points: Point for pain of neck, Houxi (SI 3) and Qiangu (SI 2).

Secondary points: Shaoze (SI 1), Zhongzhu (SJ 3), eye area and stomach area.

[Therapeutic methods]

Regular acupuncture is applied at the point for pain of neck and Houxi and Qiangu points; the bleeding therapy is applied at Zhongzhu point; and massage is performed in the eye and stomach areas.

7. Periarthritis of shoulder

[Pathogenesis and clinical manifestations]

The disease is also called frozen shoulder or Loujianfeng in Traditional Chinese Medicine, common in people of about 50 years of age. In general, it is caused by hyperplasia and adhesion of the soft tissues around the shoulder joint due to degeneration of bursas, tendons and ligaments and an aseptic infection in the joint. Important symptoms of the disease are pain and limitation of movement of the shoulder joint. In some patients, this is accompanied by muscular atrophy of the shoulder.

[Hand diagnosis]

In the area of left (right) shoulder and arm, the presence of one or several spots or patches in a white color or a white alternating blue color indicates periarthritis of shoulder with pain. The light yellow callus-like hard papule in this area indicates chronic periarthritis with adhesion after repeated inflammatory attacks.

[Selection of points]

First-choice points: Houxi (SI 3) and point for pain of shoulder.

Secondary points: Zhongzhu (SJ 3), point for pain of neck and area of left (right) shoulder and arm.

[Therapeutic methods]

Massage is performed in the area of left (right) shoulder and arm, and regular acupuncture is applied at Houxi, point for pain of shoulder, Zhongzhu, and point for pain of neck. At the same time, patients are asked to move their shoulder and arm for achieving an early improvement of the disease.

8. Strain of the lumbar muscles
[Pathogenesis and clinical manifestations]
This is a chronic injury of muscles and faciae in the lumbosacral region with persistent or intermittent attacks of lumbago and weakness of the waist, which can be exacerbated by dampness and cloudy and rainy days.

[Hand diagnosis]
In the waist area, the presence of a white patch or a light yellow callus-like papule indicates chronic lumbago with a long clinical course.

[Selection of points]
First-choice points: Point for lumbago and point of kidney.
Secondary points: Waist area and kidney area.

[Therapeutic methods]
Regular acupuncture is applied at the point for lumbago and point of kidney, and massage is performed in the waist area and kidney area. At the same time, patients are asked to move their lower back to reinforce the therapeutic effect of the treatment.

9. Prolapse of lumbar intervertebral disc
[Pathogenesis and clinical manifestations]
This is a degenerative syndrome caused by a rupture of degenerated intervertebral disc, deformity of the nucleus and fibrous ring of the disc and narrowing of intervertebral space to make the neucleus pulposus and annulus fibrosus protrusion and press the nerve roots and spinal cord. Patients may suffer from lumbago in the early stage, and then the radiating pain along the route of sciatic nerve is spread to its innervating regions, including the back of the thigh, back and side of the leg and side of the foot. Patients also show tenderness between L4 and L5 or L5 and S1, limitation of movement of the

waist and a positive Lasegue's sign.

[Hand diagnosis]

In the early stage of the disease, a papule in a red alternating with white color appears on the dark skin in the waist area. The presence of some yellowish brown or dark yellow nodules in this area indicates a long clinical course of the disease with repeated relapses. Some positive (special) signs can be found in the corresponding region of lumbar spine.

[Selection of points]

First-choice points: Point of lumbago, Houxi (SI 3) and point for pain of spine.

Secondary points: Waist area and kidney area.

[Therapeutic methods]

In the chronic stage, regular acupuncture is applied at the point for lumbago, Houxi and point for pain of spine and massage is performed in the waist area and kidney area. Patients in the acute stage should take bed rest and receive traction therapy for the lower back.

10. Heel pain

[Pathogenesis and clinical manifestations]

This is a disease with pain on the bones of the bottom of one or both heels, which may be exacerbated after standing and walking. It is common in women of 40-60 years old, particularly in the obese patients. The disease with an insidious onset and progress is caused by chronic trauma or deformity of the foot.

[Hand diagnosis]

Some light yellow or yellowish brown spots can be found on both sides of the upper and middle two-thirds of the proximal segment of ring finger.

[Selection of points]

First-choice point: Point for pain of heel.

Secondary point: Kidney area.

[Therapeutic methods]

Regular acupuncture is applied at the point for pain of heel and massage is performed in the kidney area. At the same time, patients should take a hot water bath of their feet in a 5 percent vinegar solution for 20-30 minutes, once a day for five days as a therapeutic course.

11. Sprain of the ankle joint

[Pathogenesis and clinical manifestations]

This is the most common joint sprain in comparison with sprains of all other joints in the body. It is usually caused by falling down from the heights or a sudden inversion of the ankle joint while walking over an uneven road pavement, jumping up with the lateral aspect of the foot to touch the ground or missing a step when going downstairs. Patients may have difficulty walking as they suffer from pain and swelling around the bruised joint.

[Hand diagnosis]

One or several spots or patches in a red alternating with white color may appear on both sides of the middle one third of the proximal segment of ring finger. The bluish white patch indicates a severe injury.

[Selection of points]

First-choice point: Point for pain of medial malleolus.

Secondary points: Corresponding area and liver area.

[Therapeutic methods]

Regular acupuncture is applied at the point for pain of medial malleolus, and massage is performed in the corresponding area on the palm and liver area. According to the theory of Traditional Chinese Medicine, the liver can control how an injury to the tendons develops.

12. Chronic appendicitis

[Pathogenesis and clinical manifestations]

This is a chronic inflammation in the cavity of the appendix, caused by an infection of multiple strains of bacteria and the stricture and obstruction of the appendiceal cavity by fecal matter, parasites and food debris. An important symptom of the disease is pain in right lower abdomen with nausea, vomiting, poor appetite and constipation or diarrhea.

[Hand diagnosis]

A yellow papule appears in the central region of the area of lower abdomen.

[Selection of points]

First-choice points: Point of large intestine and Hegu (LI 4).

Secondary points: Point of Sanjiao and area of lower abdomen.

[Therapeutic methods]

Regular acupuncture is applied at the point of large intestine, Hegu and point of Sanjiao. Massage is applied in the area of lower abdomen.

13. Prolapse of the rectum

[Pathogenesis and clinical manifestations]

The disease is also called prolapse of anus with the intestinal mucosa or intestinal walls of rectum and part of sigmoid colon dropping out of the anus. It is common in aged people, children and women after multiple labors. The important symptom of the disease is the prolapse of rectum after bowel movement with a tenesmus and distension sensation in the anus. In mild type, the prolapsed contents can be spontaneously replaced, but the prolapsed contents must be replaced with hand in severe type. The rectum may also drop out of the anus after cough, sneezing, walking and physical exertion. The patients of severe type also suffer from a constant desire to defecate, distending pain in the lower abdomen and frequent urination.

[Hand diagnosis]

Some spots and nodules in a red alternating with white color are present in the rectum area and few dark red fine stripes appear underneath the skin in the anus area.

[Selection of points]

First choice points: Rectum area, Hegu (LI 4) and Laogong (PC 8).

Secondary points: Anus area, stomach area and kidney area.

[Therapeutic methods]

Regular acupuncture is applied at Hegu and Laogong points; massage with thumb is performed in the rectum, anus, stomach and kidney areas; and the magnetic plates are applied in the rectum, anus and kidney areas.

[Remarks]

Chinese herbs to replenish qi of Zhongjiao (spleen and stomach) and kidney can produce a double effect if prescribed with hand acupuncture therapy, because prolapse of the rectum is thought in Traditional Chinese Medicine to be caused by a deficiency and decent of Zhongjiao qi.

14. External humeral epicondylitis

[Pathogenesis and clinical manifestations]

The disease is also called tennis elbow, due to damage at the origin of the radial extensor muscle of wrist, caused by inadequate exertion to rotate the forearm. The important symptom of the disease is pain around the lateral humeral epicondyle and humeroradial joint. The pain can be exacerbated by forcefully making a fist and rotating the forearm. Physical examination can clearly show the tender spots on the external humeral epicondyle, humeroradial joint and anterior border of the head of radius.

[Hand diagnosis]

A white color or a white alternating with blue color can be seen over the lower part of the area of shoulder and arm. Some small blue blood vessels are present underneath the skin and a light yellow callus-like papule appears on the skin in the area of shoulder and arm.

[Selection of points]

First-choice points: Shoulder and arm point, Hegu (LI 4), Houxi (SI 3) and neck point area.

[Therapeutic methods]

Massage is performed in the above-mentioned points and area.

[Remarks]

The local blocking therapy with anesthetic drugs may be used to control an acute attack of the disease in patients with impairment of movement of the upper arm and forearm.

15. Hyperplastic spondylitis

[Pathogenesis and clinical manifestations]

The disease is also called degenerative spondylitis of the cervical and lumbar spine. X-rays may show reduction or elimination of the physiological curvature of the spinal column, apparent labial hyperplasia along vertebral borders, reduction of intervertebral spaces, and a blurred image of the zygapophyseal joints. An important symptom of the disease is a chronic aching in the cervical and lumbar spine with a radiating pain to the upper and lower limbs. This is a disease common in people over 40 years of age, caused by a congenital or acquired deformity of the spinal column, spondylitis, or trauma of the spinal column.

[Hand diagnosis]

The upper one-third of the spine area and back area is the corresponding region of the neck and cervical spine and the lower one-third of those areas is the corresponding region of the lumbar spine and sacrum. The presence of a brown or brownish black plague in those regions indicates a degenerative lesion in the corresponding portion of the spinal column.

[Selection of points]

First-choice points: Point for pain of neck, waist area and point for lumbago.

Secondary points: Houxi (SI 3), Zhongzhu (SJ 3) and Qiangu (SI 2).

[Therapeutic methods]

Regular acupuncture is applied at the point for pain of neck, point for lumbago, Houxi, Zhongzhu and Qiangu. Massage is performed in the waist area.

[Remarks]

Patients are asked to do adequate exercise for their waist and make sure to keep the area warm.

Section 3 Common Diseases of Gynecology

1. Dysmenorrhea
[Pathogenesis and clinical manifestations]

Dysmenorrhea can be divided into a primary and a secondary type with lower abdominal pain before, during or after the menstrual period. It is caused by psychological factors, hypoplasia of uterus, anteversion or retroversion of the uterus, stenosis of the uterine cervix, endocrine disturbance, pelvic and intrauterine inflammation or tumors.

[Hand diagnosis]

In women with dysmenorrhea, a bluish white or brown patch or in a red alternating with white color may be present in the area of reproductive organs.

[Selection of points]

First-choice points: Point of Mingmen and point of Sanjiao.

Secondary point: Area of reproductive organs.

[Therapeutic methods]

Regular acupuncture is applied at the point of Mingmen and point of Sanjiao, and massage is performed in the area of reproductive organs.

[Remarks]

Patients should see the gynecologists to find out the cause of their dysmenorrhea, because it may be a symptom of many gynecological diseases.

2. Profuse leukorrhea
[Pathogenesis and clinical manifestation]

The normal vaginal discharge is a white sticky fluid similar to the saliva and nasal discharge, but the discharge of leukorrhea in an extraordinarily large amount or a discharge of leukorrhea with an abnormal color, nature and smell is a disease in women. Patients may also suffer from aching in the waist and knees and other general symptoms. An infection or tumors in the female reproductive organs are common causes. Constant mechanical irritation and trauma to the vagina is an important inducing factor of the disease.

[Hand diagnosis]

In the uterus area, the presence of a red or brown patch or in a red alternating with white color indicates profuse discharge of yellow and red leukorrhea. If the skin in the uterus area is shiny, depressed and bluish white in color, the leukorrhea is profuse in amount or black in color.

[Selection of points]

First-choice points: Point of Sanjiao, point of Mingmen and point of spleen.

Secondary points: Area of reproductive organs and spleen area.

[Therapeutic methods]

Regular acupuncture is applied at the point of Sanjiao, point of Mingmen and point of spleen. Massage is performed in the area of reproductive organs and spleen area. The spleen area is selected because the spleen can control "metabolism of water and dampness in the body" and deficiency of spleen may cause diseases of menses and leukorrhea.

3. Pelvic inflammation

[Pathogenesis and clinical manifestations]

As a common gynecological disease, pelvic inflammation can be divided into an acute or chronic type. Acute pelvic inflammation may involve the uterus, oviducts and/or pelvic peritoneum. Patients usually suffer from fever, lower abdominal pain, profuse leukorrhea and irregular menses. In weak patients, chronic pelvic inflammation is a protracted disease derived from an acute inflammation from failure to treat the disease in time. Patients often suffer from a tenesmus and distending sensation with pain in the lower abdomen, aching in the lumbar and sacral regions, profuse leukorrhea and disturbed menstrual cycles. Gynecological examination may show signs of a fixed uterus.

[Hand diagnosis]

The hand diagnosis of the disease is complicated and varied in accordance with the location of the lesion. In acute pelvic inflammation, a large bluish white patch or in a red alternating with white color is present in the whole area of the reproductive organs. If the inflammation is limited to the uterus, a bluish white patch is present in the uterus area. The presence of a papule in a red alternating with white color in the left or right part of the area of reproductive organs indicates an inflammation of the left and right appendage respectively.

[Selection of points]

First-choice points: Point of Mingmen, point of Sanjiao and point for lumbago.

Secondary points: Point for high fever, area of reproductive organs, liver area and spleen area.

[Therapeutic methods]

Regular acupuncture is applied at the point of Mingmen, point of Sanjiao, point for lumbago and point for high fever; and massage is performed in the area of reproductive organs, liver area and spleen area.

[Remarks]

In the acute stage of a severe inflammation, the usual gynecological therapy should be applied to patients in coordination with hand acupuncture to avoid delay of treatment and mismanagement.

4. Chronic cervicitis

[Pathogenesis and clinical manifestations]

This is a chronic inflammation of the uterine cervix caused by infectious pathogens hidden in the mucosa of the cervical canal — difficult to be detected and completely removed. As a common gynecological disease, chronic cervicitis also can be caused by local trauma and endocrine disturbances. Patients may suffer from the discharge of profuse, sticky and occasionally purulent leukorrhea, pain in the lumbar and sacral region, pain and a distending and tenesmus sensation in the lower abdomen, intercourse pain and infertility. A gynecological examination may show ulceration, mucosal hyperplasia, congestion and hypertrophy of the uterine cervix. The disease should be timely and effectively cured because it may cause development of cervical carcinoma.

[Hand diagnosis]

The presence of some white or yellow spots in the lower part of the area of reproductive organs and near the wrist crease indicates adnexitis or cervical ulceration.

[Selection of points]

First-choice points: Point of Mingmen and point of Sanjiao.

Secondary points: Area of reproductive organs and area of lumbar spine.

[Therapeutic methods]

Regular acupuncture is applied at the point of Mingmen and point of Sanjiao; and massage is performed in the area of the reproductive organs and the area of the lumbar spine.

5. Uterine contraction pain after childbirth

[Pathogenesis and clinical manifestations]

This is a postpartum pain of the lower abdomen due to an uncoordinated contraction of a localized portion of the uterus in 1-2 days after childbirth. It is common in women who have had many births and after a precipitate labor. A mild attack needs no treatment. A severe attack is paroxysmal in nature and can be exacerbated by breastfeeding. During an attack of uterine contraction pain, the uterus becomes spastic and hardened, and the discharge of lochia is increased.

[Hand diagnosis]

Some bluish white spots appear in the uterus area and a blue patch is present in the liver area.

[Selection of points]

First-choice points: Point of Mingmen and Wailaogong (EX-UE 8).

Secondary points: Area of reproductive organs and liver area.

[Therapeutic methods]

Regular acupuncture is applied at the point of Mingmen and Wailaogong point; massage is performed in the area of reproductive organs and liver area.

6. Dysfunctional uterine bleeding

[Pathogenesis and clinical manifestations]

This is an extraordinarily profuse bleeding of the uterine mucosa caused by an endocrine disturbance in patients without organic lesions in their reproductive organs. It can be divided into the ano-vulatory and ovulatory type. The former type is common in patients in either the adolescent or menopausal period with disturbance of ovulation; and the latter type is a disease in patients of childbearing age with dysfunction of corpus luteum. Important symptoms of the disease are disturbed menses, increased menstrual flow, prolonged menstrual period or spotting of uterine blood, together with anemic symptoms, such as a pale complexion, heart palpitations and general weakness of the body.

[Hand diagnosis]

A dark red color appears in the area of reproductive organs of women, which may spread to the wrist crease.

[Selection of points]

First-choice points: Area of reproductive organs, point of spleen and point of Mingmen.

Secondary points: Area of Sanjiao and point of liver.

[Therapeutic methods]

Regular acupuncture is applied at the point of spleen, point of Mingmen and point of liver; massage is performed in the area of reproductive organs and area of Sanjiao; and magnetic plates are applied in the area of reproductive organs and area of Sanjiao.

[Remarks]

Menopausal women with repeated uterine bleeding need a gy-necological examination to rule out any organic lesion. If hand acupuncture therapy alone is ineffective, some hemostatic and antishock therapies should be adopted in time to control uterine bleeding.

7. Hysteromyoma

[Pathogenesis and clinical manifestations]

This is a common benign tumor of the reproductive system in women between the ages of 30-50 years. It may be caused by excessive estrogen. The clinical manifestations of the disease are varied according to the location, size, speed of growth and complications of the tumor. Its common symptoms are uterine bleeding, abdominal mass, profuse leukorrhea, infertility and other symptoms due to the pressure of the tumor on its neighboring structures.

[Hand diagnosis]

White, yellow or dark brown round nodules are present in the area of reproductive organs.

[Selection of points]

First-choice points: Area of reproductive organs, liver area and point of spleen.

Secondary points: Point of Mingmen, area of Sanjiao and spleen area.

[Therapeutic methods]

Regular acupuncture is applied at the point of spleen and point of Mingmen; and massage is performed in the area of reproductive organs, liver area, area of Sanjiao and spleen area.

8. Amenorrhea

[Pathogenesis and clinical manifestations]

The disease can be divided into a primary and secondary type. In the primary type, patients have not menarche after 18 years of age. In the secondary type, patients between menarche and menopause who are not pregnant or breastfeeding have their normal menses interrupted for more than 3 months. Amenorrhea may be caused by maldevelopment of the uterus and ovary, endocrine dysfunction and psychological factors.

[Hand diagnosis]

The skin in the area of the reproductive organs is smooth, shiny, bluish white in color and scattered with some pits.

[Selection of points]

First-choice points: Area of reproductive organs, kidney area and point of Mingmen.

Secondary points: Point of kidney and liver area.

[Therapeutic methods]

Regular acupuncture is applied at the point of Mingmen and point of kidney; massage is performed in the area of reproductive organs, kidney area and liver area; and magnetic plate can also be applied in the liver area.

Section 4. Common Pediatric Diseases

1. Persistent pneumonia in children

[Pathogenesis and clinical manifestations]

This is a chronic infection of the lung in children caused by ineffective or delayed treatment for acute pneumonia or due to reduced immunity and weak physique of the patients. The infection may last for several months and resist various treatments. Patients may suffer from high fever, cough, dyspnea, asthma, poor appetite and increased white blood cell count.

[Hand diagnosis]

The brown patches, small pits or hard nodules are present in the area of left (right) lung and some spots in a red alternating white color appear in the lung area and near the central portion of the trachea area.

[Selection of points]

First-choice points: Yuji (LU 10), Shaoshang (LU 11), point for high fever and point of lung.

Secondary points: Lung area, trachea area and spleen area.

[Therapeutic methods]

Quick acupuncture is applied at Yuji, point for high fever and point of lung with needles immediately removed away from those points; bleeding therapy is applied at Shaoshang point; and massage is performed in the lung, trachea and spleen areas.

2. Diarrhea in children

[Pathogenesis and clinical manifestations]

As a common pediatric disease (also called children's indigestion) of summer and autumn in children below 2 years old, this disease is caused by inadequate feeding and bacterial or viral infection. Patients usually suffer from an increase of bowel activity to void thin or watery stool with a sour and putrefied bad smell. In serious cases, the diarrhea may cause dehydration, acidosis and disturbance of electrolytes. Patients with chronic diarrhea may develop poor nutrition and retardation of growth.

[Hand diagnosis]

A patch in a white color or few spots in a red alternating white color are present in the area of lower abdomen.

[Selection of points]

First-choice points: Hegu (LI 4), point for diarrhea and point of large intestine.

Secondary points: Point for pain of stomach and intestine, area of lower abdomen and spleen area.

[Therapeutic methods]

Quick acupuncture is applied at Hegu, point for diarrhea and point of large intestine with needles removed away immediately; massage is performed at the point for pain of stomach and intestine and in the area of lower abdomen and spleen area.

3. Asthma in children

[Pathogenesis and clinical manifestations]

This is an allergic disease of children with repeated attacks of coughing and wheezing in the autumn and winter. The onset of the disease may be prompt or gradual, and babies may have a runny nose and mild cough before the attack. In older babies, the attacks often burst out promptly at night or in the early morning with a fit of coughing and a high-pitched wheezing noise in the throat after a prolonged exhalation of air. The attack may be induced by many allergens, such as cold air, pollens, fur, paint, fish and shrimp. Patients often have a family history of the disease and a history of allergies.

[Hand diagnosis]

A white papule is present in the trachea area.

[Selection of points]

First-choice points: Yuji (LU 10), point of lung and Laogong (PC 8).

Secondary points: Trachea area and lung area.

[Therapeutic methods]

Quick acupuncture is applied at Yuji, point of lung and Laogong with needles pulled away immediately; massage is performed in the trachea and lung areas.

[Remarks]

Besides hand acupuncture therapy, some spasmolytic drugs should be prescribed to babies with prompt and severe attacks. Antibiotics should be administered to those with infection in their respiratory tract.

4. Convulsions in children

[Pathogenesis and clinical manifestations]

Convulsion is called Jingfeng in Traditional Chinese Medicine, and a convulsion in children below 5 years old is an acute disease due to organic lesions or functional disturbance of their nervous system. An attack of convulsions is often caused by high fever, infection of the central nervous system, toxic bacillary dysentery, dehydration or disturbance of electrolytes. The chief clinical symptoms are sudden loss of consciousness and general or local convulsions with both eyes staring upward or deviated to the side. In general, a seizure may last for several seconds or a few minutes, but it may repeatedly relapse and even persist for a very long period in critical patients.

[Hand diagnosis]

A bluish white or bluish purple patch or some blue engorged blood vessels underneath the skin may appear in the head area.

[Selection of points]

First-choice points: Point to control epilepsy and point for emergent treatment.

Secondary point: Zhongchong (PC 9).

[Therapeutic methods]

Quick acupuncture is applied at the point to control epilepsy and point for emergent treatment with needles immediately pulled away; bleeding therapy is applied at Zhongchong point.

[Remarks]

Critical babies with severe seizures that cannot be controlled by this treatment should be transferred to a general hospital immediately for an emergency rescue.

5. Anorexia in children

[Pathogenesis and clinical manifestation]

Anorexia in children is called "Ganji" in the Traditional Chinese Medicine. It is a common disease of children ages 1-6 years. Poor appetite and even refusal to take food for a long time is its chief clinical manifestation. Babies may also suffer from abdominal distension and pathologic leanness with nausea and vomiting often caused by a forceful or overfull feeding. Fundamental causes that impair digestive function are children's dietary preference, irregular food habits and greediness for snacks in spoiled children.

[Hand diagnosis]

The skin in the stomach area is shiny, depressed and white in color and a dark red patch may appear in this area.

[Selection of points]

First-choice points: Sifeng (EX-UE 10) points.

Secondary points: Stomach area, spleen area and area of large intestine.

[Therapeutic methods]

After four Sifeng points of each hand are pricked with a needle, some yellowish white fluid is squeezed out from the pinholes; massage is performed in the stomach area, spleen area and area of large intestine.

6. Bed-wetting in children

[Pathogenesis and clinical manifestations]

This is a common disease of children above 3 years of age with frequent bed-wetting (incontinence of urine) in their sleep at night. They become aware that they have wet the bed only after waking up in the morning. The frequency of bed-wetting may be one to several times per night and the children also show tiredness, pale complexion and leanness of body.

[Hand diagnosis]

A white or dark gray papule is present in the bladder area and some white spots appear in the kidney area.

[Selection of points]

First-choice points: Bladder area, point for bed-wetting and point of Sanjiao.

Secondary points: Kidney area, heart area and Zhongchong (PC 9).

[Therapeutic methods]

Quick acupuncture is applied at the point for bed-wetting and point of Sanjiao with needles immediately removed away; bleeding therapy is applied at Zhongchong point to squeeze out 2−3 drops of blood; and massage with thumb is performed in the bladder, kidney and heart areas.

[Remarks]

Abnormal urination in some children is related to nervousness, shamefulness and overfatigue, therefore, some explanation and comfort should be made to relieve their mental pressures.

7. Poor nutrition in children

[Pathogenesis and clinical manifestations]

This is a common disease of infants and young children below 3 years of age with chronic nutritional and metabolic disturbances due to prolonged inadequate feeding, diet preference, and digestive and some absorptive disorders caused by intestinal parasites and diseases of the digestive system. Patients may show sallow or pale complexion, pathologic leanness, dryness of skin and hair, poor appetite, abdominal distension, fatigue and weakness, restlessness, crying and fear at night and retardation of intelligence and locomotive functions.

[Hand diagnosis]

The skin in the stomach and spleen areas is white, shiny and depressed; one or some red or dark red spots and patches are present in the lower one-third of the abdomen area.

[Selection of points]

First-choice points: Stomach area, spleen area, Hegu (LI 4) and Sifeng (EX-UE 10).

Secondary points: Heart area and lower one-third of abdomen area.

[Therapeutic methods]

Quick acupuncture is applied at Hegu point with needle immediately removed away; bleeding therapy is applied at Sifeng points of both hands to squeeze 1-2 drops of pale yellow fluid; and massage with thumb is performed in the stomach area, spleen area, area of lower one-third of abdomen and heart area.

[Remarks]

A good dietary habit should be established for babies to avoid a diet preference. A routine examination of stool should be made regularly to rule out and treat in time intestinal parasites.

8. Cerebral dysgenesis

[Pathogenesis and clinical manifestations]

This is a disease of infants with retarded development of the brain with its functions due to some hereditary factors, labor trauma, asphyxia of prolonged labor, intracranial infection, and some diseases suffered by the mother during her pregnancy. Important clinical manifestations are a disturbance of intelligence and various neurological symptoms, such as mental deficiency, slow movement, rigid paralysis of lower limbs, a scissors gait, seizures and failure to take care of one's daily life.

[Hand diagnosis]

Some bluish purple subcutaneous blood vessels are present in the head area.

[Selection of points]

First-choice points: Head area, Houxi (SI 3), Zhongzhu (SJ 3) and kidney area.

Secondary points: Zhongchong (PC 9) and point for epilepsy.

[Therapeutic methods]

Quick acupuncture is applied at Houxi, Zhongzhu and point for epilepsy with needles immediately removed away; bleeding therapy with a three-edged needle is applied at Zhongchong point to squeeze out 1-2 drops of blood; and massage with thumb is performed in the head and kidney areas.

Section 5　Common Diseases of Eye, Nose, Ear, Oral Cavity and Throat

1. Myopia

[Pathogenesis and clinical manifestations]

This is an eye abnormality. The image of the parallel light from an object three meters away from the eye is focused in front of the retina after refraction through the refracting apparatus of the eye. Myopia can be divided into a true and false type. True myopia is caused by an abnormally elongated optic axis or increased refractive index of the cornea; false myopia is caused by a spasm of the ciliary muscle and an increase of convexity of the lens caused by eye fatigue or a bad habit such as reading books to close to the face. False myopia may turn into the true type, if it is not checked and corrected in time.

[Hand diagnosis]

The presence of an oblique line (or a depressed oblique band with its upper border wider than the lower one) drawn from the lateral border of the eye area (the crease between index and middle finger or between middle and ring finger) to the area of nose and mouth indicates myopia. The occurrence of a grayish white patch in the eye area is also an indication of myopia.

[Selection of points]

First-choice points: Point of liver, point for pain of eye and Yemen (SJ 2).

Secondary points: Liver area and eye area.

[Therapeutic methods]

Regular acupuncture is applied at the point for pain of eye and Yemen point; and massage is performed in the liver and eye areas.

2. Hordeolum (sty)

[Pathogenesis and clinical manifestations]

This is an acute infection of the eyelid glands caused by pyogenic bacteria. In the early stage, a hard nodule with local redness, swelling, pain and tenderness appears on the eyelid that turns into a yellow pustule a few days later. The pustule will rupture and the sufferings of pain, redness and swelling may gradually be relieved in about one week.

[Hand diagnosis]

A white patch or papule occurs in the eye area with the size of the patch in proportion to that of the infection.

[Selection of points]

First-choice points: Yemen (SJ 2), Shangyang (LI 1) and point of liver.

Secondary points: Eye area and liver area.

[Therapeutic methods]

Regular acupuncture is applied at Yemen and point of liver; bleeding therapy is applied at Shangyang point; and massage is performed in the liver and eye areas.

3. Conjunctivitis

[Pathogenesis and clinical manifestations]

This is an acute inflammation of the conjunctiva of the eye commonly known as "red eye disease," caused by chemical and physical irritation or an invasion of microbial pathogens. It is highly transmissible. The onset of the disease is prompt, and its chief symptoms are congestion and swelling of the bulbar conjunctiva, swelling of the eyelids, increase of excretion, burning sensation and photophobia of the eye. Patients with chronic conjunctivitis may suffer from itching, a burning sensation, dryness, a sensation of something in the eye and tiredness of the eye.

[Hand diagnosis]

A red color in the eye area indicates acute conjunctivitis; and a white, yellow or yellowish brown color in this area indicates chronic conjunctivitis.

[Selection of points]

First-choice points: Sanjian (LI 3), Yemen (SJ 2) and point for pain of eye.

Secondary points: Eye area and liver area.

[Therapeutic methods]

Regular acupuncture is applied at Sanjian, Yemen and point for pain of eye; massage is performed in the eye and liver areas.

4. Trachoma

[Pathogenesis and clinical manifestations]

This is a chronic infectious disease of the eye caused by chlamydia. In the early stage, patients may have no symptoms, but at the acute or deteriorated stage, they may suffer from a friction sensation in the eye, photophobia, tearing and increased excretions of the eye. An ophthalmologic examination may show swelling of the eyelids, conjunctival congestion, follicles all over the upper and lower fornices of eye and edema of corneal epithelium. In the late stages, vision may be impaired due to dryness of the eyeball, entropion and trichiasis.

[Hand diagnosis]

A white papule or some red spots may appear in the eye area.

[Selection of points]

First-choice points: Eye area, Yemen (SJ 2) and point of liver.

Secondary points: Liver area and Hegu (LI 4).

[Therapeutic methods]

Regular acupuncture is applied at Yemen, Hegu and point of liver; massage with thumb is performed to press the eye and liver areas; and magnetic plates are applied in the eye and liver areas.

[Remarks]

Patients should be taught proper eye hygiene and avoid spicy and greasy foods. Surgical correction is necessary in patients with entropion and trichiasis.

5. Electric ophthalmitis

[Pathogenesis and clinical manifestations]

This is a common occupational disease of the eye with inflammation of conjunctiva and cornea caused by irradiation of ultraviolet light from a strong light source. In patients with a mild case, the clinical symptoms include the sense of something in the eye, mild dryness and pain in both eyes. In a severe attack, patients may suffer from burning pain in the face and eyes, shedding of hot tears, photophobia, spasms of the eyelids with difficulty to open their eyes, dense spotty or patchy exfoliation of the iris, turbid anterior chamber fluid and contraction of the pupils. The symptoms mentioned above may sustain for 6-14 hours and even to 48 hours in severe cases.

[Hand diagnosis]

A red color appears in the eye area.

[Selection of points]

First-choice points: Eye area, Hegu (LI 4), point for pain of eye and Yemen (SJ 2).

Secondary points: Liver area and Zhongchong (PC 9).

[Therapeutic methods]

Regular acupuncture is applied at the point for pain of eye, Yemen and Hegu points; bleeding therapy with three-edged needle is applied at Zhongchong point to squeeze out 2-3 drops of blood; and massage with thumb is performed to press the eye and liver areas.

6. Keratitis

[Pathogenesis and clinical manifestations]

This is an inflammation of the cornea caused by the microbial infection, trauma or chemical and physical irritation with a marked sense of something in the eye, photophobia, tearing and pain in the eye. Patients may suffer from turbidity of the cornea and impairment of vision after repeated attacks.

[Hand diagnosis]

A red color in present in the eye area and a red or dark red color appears in the liver area.

[Selection of points]

First-choice points: Point for pain of eye, Shangyang (LI 1) and Zhongchong (PC 9).

Secondary points: Liver area and eye area.

[Therapeutic methods]

Regular acupuncture is applied at the point for pain of eye; bleeding therapy is applied at Shangyang and Zhongchong points to squeeze out few drops of blood; and massage is performed in the liver and eye areas.

7. Retinal periphlebitis

[Pathogenesis and clinical manifestations]

This is an eye disease with inflammation of the external sheath of retinal veins or in the perivenous spaces to cause venous thrombosis or rupture of veins with retinal hemorrhage. The chief symptoms of the disease are a sudden impairment of vision and accumulation of blood in the vitreous body of both eyes one after another. A disease with repeated relapses and with male youths the most susceptible to it, retinal periphlebitis is also called juvenile recurrent hemorrhage of retina and vitreous body. In the early stages, patients may have no symptoms besides myopsis, but a diagnosis can be made if the funduscopic examination shows a white sheath around the retinal veins and some hemorrhagic spots on the retina.

[Hand diagnosis]

Some fresh red, dark red or dark gray spots and blue subcutaneous engorged blood vessels are present in the eye area.

[Selection of points]

First-choice points: Point for pain of eye, point of liver and Shixuan (EX-UE 11) points.

Secondary points: Liver area and eye area.

[Therapeutic methods]

Regular acupuncture is applied at the point for pain of eye and point of liver; bleeding therapy is applied at Shixuan points; and massage is performed in the liver and eye areas.

8. Allergic rhinitis

[Pathogenesis and clinical manifestations]

This is an allergic reaction of nasal mucosa with paroxysmal attacks of itching in the nose, repeated sneezing, profuse runny nose, headache and tearing caused by the inhalation of pollen, smoke and dust or irritation by cold or hot wind. The attack usually lasts for only several minutes, but it may persistently linger over years in some stubborn cases.

[Hand diagnosis]

The skin in the nose area is smooth, depressed and gray in color.

[Selection of points]

First-choice points: Hegu (LI 4), Erjian (LI 2) and point of lung.

Secondary points: Nose area and lung area.

[Therapeutic methods]

Regular acupuncture is applied at Hegu, Erjian and point of lung and massage is performed in the nose and lung areas.

9. Atrophic rhinitis

[Pathogenesis and clinical manifestations]

As a chronic rhinitis of unknown cause, the atrophy of nasal mucosa is a particular lesion of the disease. In severe cases, the nasal periosteum and bones are also involved to cause shrinkage of the nasal conchae and expansion of the nasal cavity. The chief symptoms of the disease are dryness in the nose and nasal obstruction. In severe cases, some pus crusts that are foul smelling form in the nasal cavity.

[Hand diagnosis]

The skin in the nose area is depressed, scattered with fine striae, and in an uneven dark gray color.

[Selection of points]

First-choice points: Shaoshang (LU 11), Hegu (LI 4) and point of lung.

Secondary points: Nose area and lung area.

[Therapeutic methods]

Regular acupuncture is applied at Shaoshang, Hegu and point of lung; and massage is performed in the nose and lung areas.

10. Chronic sinusitis

[Pathogenesis and clinical manifestations]

This is a common nasal disease in patients of any age. As a chronic disease derived from acute rhinitis, it may linger for years and resist treatment. Patients may suffer from purulent nasal discharge, nasal obstruction, reduction of the ability to smell, tenderness beside the nose, vertigo, poor memory and a unilateral dull pain in the head that may be exacerbated during physical exertion or lowering the head.

[Hand diagnosis]

A vertical callus-like prominence in a dark red color is present in the center of the nose area.

[Selection of points]

First-choice points: Hegu (LI 4), point of lung and Erjian (LI 2).

Secondary points: Nose area and lung area.

[Therapeutic methods]

Regular acupuncture is applied at Hegu, point of lung and Erjian point and massage is performed in the nose and lung areas.

11. Nasal bleeding

[Pathogenesis and clinical manifestations]

This is a common clinical symptom caused by external trauma, emotional disturbance or hot and dry weather. The bleeding is usually brought on in the spring and autumn and in children and youths.

In severe cases, the bleeding is profuse and difficult to control.

[Hand diagnosis]

A blue or purplish red subcutaneous blood vessel passes through the nose area.

[Selection of points]

First-choice points: Nose area, Hegu (LI 4), Shaoshang (LU 11) and lung area.

Secondary point: Point of lung.

[Therapeutic methods]

Regular acupuncture is applied at Hegu and point of lung; bleeding therapy with a three-edged needle is applied at Shaoshang point to squeeze out 2-3 drops of blood; and massage with thumb is performed to press the nose area and bilateral lung areas.

[Remarks]

Besides the hand acupuncture therapy, other hemostatic therapies must be adopted to control the profuse nasal bleeding.

12. Foreign body sensation in throat

[Pathogenesis and clinical manifestations]

This is a common disease of the throat caused by emotional disturbance, mental nervousness or overfatigue. The disease is common in women of middle age and it may come on in any season of a year. The chief symptom of the disease is a sensation of having something in the throat, same as the ant crawling or obstruction of the throat by a ball. The sensation becomes more apparent during an attempt to swallow (without swallowing food or drink), although there is no obstacle to swallowing food. A laryngoscopic examination and fluoroscopy with barium meal show no abnormality.

[Hand diagnosis]

Some white or pink spots are present in the mouth area.

[Selection of points]

First-choice points: Mouth area, Shaoshang (LU 11) and Yuji (LU 10).

Secondary points: Liver area and point of throat.

[Therapeutic methods]

Regular acupuncture is applied at Shaoshang, Yuji and point of throat; and massage with thumb is applied to press the mouth and liver areas.

[Remarks]

The psychotherapy is useful to relieve the mental pressure of patients and improve the therapeutic effect of the treatment.

13. Acute tonsillitis

[Pathogenesis and clinical manifestations]

This is an acute nonspecific infection of palatal tonsils caused by hemolytic streptococcus B and other pyogenic bacteria, such as staphylococcus and streptococcus viridans. The onset of the disease is prompt with general malaise, chills, high fever with a body temperature possibly over 40 C, headache, aching in the neck and back, poor appetite, sore throat with exaggerated pain when swallowing, and enlargement and tenderness of the submaxillary lymph nodes.

[Hand diagnosis]

The holographic area of the tonsils on the hand lies just above the intersection of the extended midline of middle finger and the emotion line. Some fresh red or flushing red spots are present in this area in the patient of acute tonsillitis.

[Selection of points]

First-choice points: Guanchong (SJ 1), Yemen (SJ 2), Yangchi (SJ 4), point for high fever and point of tonsil.

Secondary points: Lung area, mouth area and head area.

[Therapeutic methods]

Regular acupuncture is applied at Yemen, Yangchi, point for high fever and point of tonsil; bleeding therapy is applied at Guanchong point and also at Shixuan (EX-UE 11) and Dazhui (DU 14) in patients with high fever; and massage is performed in the lung, mouth and head areas.

14. Acute pharyngitis

[Pathogenesis and clinical manifestations]

Different from primary acute pharyngitis caused by the infection of hemolytic streptococcus, secondary pharyngitis in most patients is derived from acute rhinitis or caused by an addiction to smoking or alcoholic drink. The common symptoms of the disease are pain and dryness in the throat and hoarseness of voice, but patients with severe acute pharyngitis may suffer from chills, fever, headache, aching of limbs and pain in the throat when swallowing.

[Hand diagnosis]

The holographic area of the throat on the hand lies slightly above and beside the intersection of the extended midline of middle finger and the emotion line. In the acute stages of the disease, some scattered white spots or in a red alternating with white color are present in this area but in the chronic stage, some yellow or dark red nodules are visible in this area. In chronic patients with acute exacerbation, some white or red spots are scattered among the yellow nodules.

[Selection of points]

First-choice points: Point of throat, Yuji (LU 10), Guanchong (SJ 1) and Shaoshang (LU 11).

Secondary points: Hegu (LI 4), Zhongzhu (SJ 3), mouth area and lung area.

[Therapeutic methods]

Regular acupuncture is applied at the point of throat, Yuji, Hegu and Zhongzhu points; bleeding therapy is applied at Guanchong and Shaoshang points; and massage is performed in the mouth and lung areas.

15. Toothache

[Pathogenesis and clinical manifestations]

This is a common symptom of dental diseases, such as caries, pulpitis and periodontal diseases. It may occur in any season and attack patients of any age. The pain may be paroxysmal and sharp or continuous and dull in nature and it may be exacerbated at night or by the stimulation of cold, hot, sour or sweet food and drink. The toothache is often accompanied with headache, thirst, looseness of teeth, sour taste and bad breath.

[Hand diagnosis]

The presence of some white spots or small patches on certain parts of the tooth area indicates inflammation and pain of the corresponding teeth. The presence of some dark yellow or yellowish brown nodules or papules in the tooth area indicates chronic inflammation or caries of the corresponding teeth. They also may indicate that the corresponding teeth have been filled.

[Selection of points]

First-choice points: Point for toothache, Hegu (LI 4) and Erjian (LI 2).

Secondary points: Tooth area, stomach area and mouth area.

[Therapeutic methods]

Regular acupuncture is applied at the point for toothache, Hegu and Erjian points; and massage is performed in the tooth, stomach and mouth areas.

16. Tinnitus and deafness

[Pathogenesis and clinical manifestations]

The tinnitus is a symptom of auditory disturbance with a high-pitched and low-pitched noise in the ear. Tinnitus with high-pitched noise is caused by organic lesions in the auditory system; tinnitus with low-pitched noise is due to a dysfunction of the auditory system. A mild type of deafness is known as hard-of-hearing while a severe type is real deafness. Both types may coexist simultaneously.

[Hand diagnosis]

The skin in the area of left (right) ear is depressed. Some small, blue and engorged subcutaneous veins are visible in this area that represent nervous tinnitus or deafness and indicate that patients are sensitive to high-pitched sound. Thick and engorged subcutaneous blood vessels in this area indicate tinnitus or deafness in patients sensitive to low-pitched sound.

[Selection of points]

First-choice points: Shangyang (LI 1), Qiangu (SI 2), Houxi (SI 3) and Yemen (SJ 2).

Secondary points: Area of left (right) ear, liver area and kidney area.

[Therapeutic methods]

Regular acupuncture is applied at Qiangu, Houxi and Yemen points; bleeding therapy applied at Shangyang point can produce a good result to cure acute tinnitus and deafness; and massage is performed in the area of left (right) ear, liver area and kidney area.

17. Inner ear vertigo

[Pathogenesis and clinical manifestations]

The disease of unknown causes is also called Meniere's syndrome or labyrinthine hydrops with dysfunction of the vegetative nervous system, accumulation of fluid in the membranous labyrinth and vestibular disorders due to allergic reaction, metabolic disturbance of water and electrolytes, and spasms of blood vessels in the inner ear. A chief symptom of the disease is a paroxysmal attack of vertigo with nausea, vomiting, pale complexion, clear consciousness, tinnitus, deafness and a sensation of fullness in the ear. The attack may last for several minutes or a few hours; it may suddenly disappear or gradually subside. Most patients also suffer from continuous tinnitus and impairment of hearing between the attacks.

[Hand diagnosis]

The skin in the area of left (right) ear is bright white in color and swollen due to local edema. Some small blue engorged veins may appear underneath the skin.

[Selection of points]

First-choice points: Houxi (SI 3), Zhongzhu (SJ 3), Shangyang (LI 1) and Hegu (LI 4).

Secondary points: Area of left (right) ear, head area and stomach area.

[Therapeutic methods]

Regular acupuncture is applied at Houxi, Zhongzhu, Hegu and Shangyang points and massage is performed in the area of left (right) ear, head area and stomach area.

18. Supraorbital neuralgia

[Pathogenesis and clinical manifestations]

This is a common ophthalmologic disease with local pain at the supraorbital notch which is the junction of the medial one-third and lateral two-thirds of the superior orbital border. During an attack of neuralgia, patients suffer from localized pain in this region that radiates to the forehead, so it is also called pain of the Meilenggu (supraorbital bone). Patients also suffer from a dull pain in the eyeball, eye fatigue, vertigo, nausea and vomiting; but they have no organic lesions of the eye. The visual acuity and eye pressure is normal. Tenderness at the supraorbital notch can be detected.

[Hand diagnosis]

The skin of the eye area and head area on the hand is white in color, and a small blue blood vessel passes through those two areas.

[Selection of points]

First-choice points: Point for pain of eye, Sanjian (LI 3) and Yemen (SJ 2).

Secondary points: Point for pain of forehead, head area, eye area and liver area.

[Therapeutic methods]

Regular acupuncture is applied at the point for pain of eye, point for pain of forehead, Sanjian and Yemen points and massage is performed in the head, eye and liver areas.

Section 6 Common Diseases of the Skin

1. Urticaria

[Pathogenesis and clinical manifestations]

This is a common skin disease with the folk name of Fengtuankuai caused by an allergic vascular reaction to some drugs, food, insects, parasites, infectious foci, animals and plants, as well as physical irritation. Urticaria can be divided into acute and chronic types. In an acute case, many papules of varied size and shape and in a fresh red or pale white color suddenly appear on the skin with severe itching. Although the chronic urticaria is derived from the acute type, chronic patients may suffer from less remarkable symptoms. Chronic cases may repeatedly relapse and linger for mouths or years.

[Hand diagnosis]

The presence of one or several white patches or papules at certain part of the skin area on the hand indicates the occurrence of urticaria lesions on the corresponding region of the body surface.

[Selection of points]

First-choice points: Hegu (LI 4), Laogong (PC 8), Shaoze (SI 1), Shangyang (LI 1) and Zhongzhu (SJ 3).

Secondary points: Skin area, lung area and spleen area.

[Therapeutic methods]

Regular acupuncture is applied at Hegu and Laogong points; bleeding therapy is applied at Shaoze and Shangyang points; and massage is performed in the skin, lung and spleen areas.

2. Cutaneous pruritus

[Pathogenesis and clinical manifestations]

This is a skin disease with a widely spread or localized itching but without primary skin lesions. It is common in adults and old persons as a symptom of some internal diseases or localized lesions of the skin itself. Cutaneous pruritus with paroxysmal attacks of generalized itching on the skin can be induced by alcoholic beverages, emotional disturbance and chafing of the clothes or other external irritations.

[Hand diagnosis]

Same as those mentioned in urticaria.

[Selection of points]

First-choice points: Yuji (LU 10), Hegu (LI 4), Yemen (SJ 2) and point of lung.

Secondary points: Skin area, lung area and Baxie (EX-UE 9) points.

[Therapeutic methods]

Regular acupuncture is applied at Yuji, Hegu, Yemen, Baxie and point of lung; and massage is performed in the skin and lung areas. In severe attacks, bleeding therapy applied at Shaoshang point can produce a good effect to relieve itching.

3. Herpes zoster

[Pathogenesis and clinical manifestations]

This is an inflammatory skin disease caused by varicella-zoster virus and it is called Chanyao Huodan or Chuanyaolong in Traditional Chinese Medicine. The disease usually comes on in the spring and autumn, and it does not reoccur after the first attack. The clinical symptoms of the disease are low fever, fatigue, poor appetite, and sensitivity, pain and itching of localized skin. In the early stages, irregular erythema appear over the itching skin and then several clusters of nodules varied in a size from millet to a mung bean appear on the erythema. Later on, these nodules are transformed into blisters with clear fluid and surrounded by a white inflamed halo while the nearby lymph nodes are enlarged. Skin lesions are arranged in a band along a cranial or spinal nerve on one side of the chest, back, face, neck, waist or abdomen. The skin between the vesicles is normal in appearance, but the skin covered by the lesions may become pigmented after the skin rashes subside.

[Hand diagnosis]

One or several nodules or papules of fresh red color or in a red alternating with white color are present in the skin area.

[Selection of points]

First-choice points: Zhongchong (PC 9), Shaoshang (LU 11), Yuji (LU 10) and Hegu (LI 4).

Secondary points: Point of lung, point of spleen, Shixuan (EX-UE 11), skin area, lung area, spleen area and heart area.

[Therapeutic methods]

Regular acupuncture is applied at Yuji, Hegu, point of lung and point of spleen; bleeding therapy is applied at Zhongchong, Shaoshang and Shixuan points; and massage is performed in the skin, lung, spleen and heart areas.

[Remarks]

In patients with prompt onset and severe symptoms — to clear the toxic-heat pathogen and improve the therapeutic effect of hand acupuncture therapy — cupping therapy may be applied on the skin lesions for 10 minutes following the application of plum-blossom acupuncture.

4. Eczema

[Pathogenesis and clinical manifestations]

This is a common allergic and inflammatory skin disease with rashes on the surface of the skin. Eczema may be caused by mental nervousness, insomnia, overfatigue, poor nutrition, indigestion, diseases of the stomach and intestine, parasites, metabolic disorders and endocrine dysfunction. The skin lesions can include erythema, papules, vesicles, erosion, exudation and crust formation. In the late stages, patients may have a thickened lichenoid skin lesions with deep grooves and clear-cut margins.

[Hand diagnosis]

A light brown or dark callus-like papule is present in the skin area.

[Selection of points]

First-choice points: Hegu (LI 4), point of spleen, point of lung and Shaoshang (LU 11).

Secondary points: Skin area, spleen area, lung area and corresponding regions of the body.

[Therapeutic methods]

Regular acupuncture is applied at Hegu, Shaoshang, point of spleen and point of lung; and massage is performed in the skin, spleen and lung areas and the corresponding regions.

5. Neurodermatitis

[Pathogenesis and clinical manifestations]

This is a common chronic hypertrophic skin disease of adults and it is called Niupixuan in Traditional Chinese Medicine. In the early stage, patients only feel some local itching, and then a bulging patch of densely packed red maculopapules appears after a vigorous scratching of the itching skin. The skin lesion may gradually become roughened, hypertrophic and lichenous with pigmentation as some thick striae and scales appear on the lesion. The lichenoid skin lesions with intractable itching are often symmetrically distributed on the neck, sacrum, elbow and knee.

[Hand diagnosis]

The presence of some dark yellow nodules in the skin area indicates neurodermatitis.

[Selection of points]

First-choice points: Yuji (LU 10), Laogong (PC 8), Houxi (SI 3) and point of lung.

Secondary points: Skin area, lung area and spleen area.

[Therapeutic methods]

Regular acupuncture is applied at Yuji, Laogong, Houxi and point of lung and massage is performed in the skin, lung and spleen areas.

6. Acne

[Pathogenesis and clinical manifestations]

This is an adolescent skin disease common in both male and female youths. The pinpoint or millet-like skin rashes are scattered on the face, anterior chest wall and upper back. They are multiform in appearance, including comedo, papule, pustule, nodule, cyst and scar. The clinical course of the disease is varied in length, but in most patients the skin lesions may spontaneously disappear after adolescence. Excessive secretion of androgen and microbial infection are the pathogenic factors of the disease; the intake of alcohol, a high carbohydrate and fat diet and spicy foods can exacerbate acne.

[Hand diagnosis]

One or several pink or dark red spots and patches are present in the cheek area.

[Selection of points]

First-choice points: Cheek area, Hegu (LI 4) and Zhongchong (PC 9).

Secondary points: Stomach area and lung area.

[Therapeutic methods]

Regular acupuncture is applied at Hegu point; bleeding therapy is applied with a three-edged needle at Zhongchong point to squeeze out 2-3 drops of blood; and massage with thumb is performed in the cheek, stomach and lung areas.

[Remarks]

Any oily creams or cosmetics should not be applied to the face, bowel movements should be kept regular and spicy foods should be removed from the diet.

Section 7 Diseases Due to Bodily Dysfunction

1. Insomnia

[Pathogenesis and clinical manifestations]

This is a clinical symptom with many causes. The only insomnia discussed in this section will be dysfunction of the vegetative nervous system and endocrine disturbance caused by long-standing nervousness, heavy mental stress, extreme fear, depression, strong emotional disturbance, or excessive study or work pressure in weak patients. Those suffering from insomnia find it difficult to fall asleep, easy to wake up and even more difficult to get back to sleep. They may also suffer from high irritability, fatigue, poor appetite, dizziness and a distending sensation in the head.

[Hand diagnosis]

The presence of small bluish purple subcutaneous veins and white patches around them in the head area indicates insomnia due to insufficient blood supply to the brain, increase of blood viscosity and reduction of metabolism.

[Selection of points]

First-choice points: Head area, lateral end of the interphalangeal crease of thumb and Laogong (PC 8).

Secondary points: Heart area, kidney area, area of reproductive organs, area for hypertension and area for hypotension.

[Therapeutic methods]

Massage is performed in all areas and over all points mentioned above for 20-30 minutes, once or twice a day to produce a sore, distending and pain sensation. Insomnia may be cured after treatment for three-five days.

2. Tired neck and shoulder muscles

[Pathogenesis and clinical manifestations]

This is a common syndrome with aching in muscles of the neck and shoulders caused by prolonged forward flexion of the cervical spine and a persistent stretch of those muscles by bending the neck for a long time over a desk with improper posture because the desk is too low or the posture is just poor. The disease is common in students, typists and computer and other office workers. Patients may suffer from an aching and distension in the neck, back and shoulder muscles, limitation of movement of neck and shoulder, numbness of upper arm, headache, dizziness, poor concentration of attention, low working efficiency, and eye fatigue.

[Hand diagnosis]

Some spots in a red alternating with white color and one or several light brown or brownish black patches can be found in the upper one fifth segment of the spine and back areas. A white color with blue tint or some blue subcutaneous blood vessels can be seen in the lateral part of the area of shoulder and arm.

[Selection of points]

First-choice points: The depressed regions on both sides of the upper one fifth of the spine and back areas, the proximal interphalangeal crease of index finger, and the region above the radial end (on the border between red and white skin) of the interphalangeal crease of thumb.

Secondary points: Head area, Houxi (SI 3) and area of shoulder and arm.

[Therapeutic methods]

For patients with severe pain, regular acupuncture is applied at

Houxi point, and they are asked to simultaneously move their neck to produce a good therapeutic effect. For a still better therapeutic result, massage is performed at the first-choice points, head area and area of shoulder and arm for 20-30 minutes to produce a soreness, distending sensation and pain.

3. Copiopia (eye fatigue)

[Pathogenesis and clinical manifestations]

This is a syndrome of eye fatigue caused by overuse of the eyes when driving a car, working on the computer, watching TV or staying up late. Patients want to repeatedly rub their eyes; and they also suffer from redness, swelling and discomfort of eyes with soreness, dryness and distending sensation in the eyeball, dizziness, distending sensation in brain, poor memory, poor concentration, tinnitus and vertigo.

[Hand diagnosis]

Some red spots or in a red alternating with white color are present in the eye area.

[Selection of points]

First-choice points: Point for pain of eye, Yangxi (LI 5) and Yemen (SJ 2).

Secondary points: Eye area, head area, liver area and kidney area.

[Therapeutic methods]

Regular acupuncture is applied at the point for pain of eye, Yangxi and Yemen points; massage is performed in the eye, head, liver and kidney areas; and bleeding therapy is applied at Shangyang (LI 1) point, if the eyes are red and swollen.

4. Reduction of vitality

[Pathogenesis and clinical manifestations]

This is a clinical syndrome caused by heavy work pressures, intense working and living habits, prolonged mental stress, depression, unhappiness and unsatisfactory sex. Patients may suffer from dizziness; a distending sensation in the brain; poor concentration;

insomnia; irritability; poor memory; soreness of the lower back and legs; fatigue and weakness; reduced sexual desire; tinnitus; a hot feeling in the chest, palms and soles; and night sweating.

[Hand diagnosis]

Some spots in a red alternating with white color and few small dark purple veins with bluish white sheath are visible in the head area; one or several dark red patches are present in the liver and kidney areas; and the skin in the kidney area and area of reproductive is pink or flushing red in color.

[Selection of points]

First-choice points: Head area, liver area, stomach area, kidney area and area of reproductive organs.

Secondary points: Area for fatigue, eye area and area for insomnia.

[Therapeutic methods]

Daily massage is performed in all holographic areas mentioned above for 20-30 minutes. A foot bath in salted warm water is taken for 20-30 minutes each night. The disease may be cured after the treatment is adopted for three-five days.

REFERENCES

1. Ma Zhongxue: *A Handbook of International Exchanges on Acupuncture*, Shandong Science and Technology Press, Jinan, 1992.

2. Zhang Yansheng and Chen Kangmei: *Qigong and Hand Acupuncture,* People's Physical Culture Publishing House, Beijing, 1993.

3. Liu Jianfeng: *Hand Acupuncture,* Hualing Publishing House, Beijing, 1992.

4. Zhang Daocheng: *New Edition of the Handbook of Predictions of the Book of Changes*, Shanxi People's Publishing House, Taiyuan, 1993.

5. Peng Qinghua and Zhang Wenan: *Observation Diagnosis on a Hundred Ailments, with Illustrations*, Scientific and Technological Documentation Publishing House, Beijing, 1996.

6. Yang Jizhou: *Great Compendium of Acupuncture and Moxibustion* (Ming Dynasty), People's Medical Publishing House, Beijing , 1983.

7. Zhang Yingqing: *Biological Holographic Therapy*, Shandong University Publishing House, Jinan, 1987.

8. Nanjing Institute of Traditional Chinese Medicine: *Acupuncture and Moxibustion*, Shanghai Science and Technology Press, Shanghai, 1979.

图书在版编目（CIP）数据

手针疗法 / 乔晋琳编著.
－北京: 外文出版社, 2002. 9
ISBN 7-119-03168-6

I. 手… II. 乔… III. 手针足针疗法－英文
IV. R245. 32

中国版本图书馆 CIP 数据核字（2002）第 068928 号

责任编辑	余冰清
英文责编	王增芬
封面设计	唐少文
插图绘制	李士伋
印刷监制	张国祥

外文出版 网址:
   http://www.flp.com.cn
外文出版 电子信箱:
   info@flp.com.cn
   sales@flp.com.cn

手针疗法

乔晋琳 　编著

王台 　　英译

*

©外文出版社
外文出版社出版
（中国北京百万庄大街 24 号）
邮政编码　100037
三河市汇鑫印务有限公司印刷
中国国际图书贸易总公司发行
（中国北京车公庄西路 35 号）
北京邮政信箱第 399 号　邮政编码　100044
2002 年(大 32 开)第 1 版
2002 年第 1 版第 1 次印刷
（英）
ISBN 7-119-03168-6/R. 163(外)
03000(平)
14-E-3515P